A Man's Dilemma

A Man's Dilemma

Understanding Prostate Cancer and Treatment Options

Stuart Rodney Wolk, PhD, J.D.

Writers Club Press
New York   Lincoln   Shanghai

A Man's Dilemma
Understanding Prostate Cancer and Treatment Options

Writers Club Press
an imprint of iUniverse, Inc.

iUniverse books may be ordered through booksellers or by contacting:

iUniverse
2021 Pine Lake Road, Suite 100
Lincoln, NE 68512
www.iuniverse.com
1-800-Authors (1-800-288-4677)

ISBN-13: 978-0-595-24337-2 (pbk)
ISBN-13: 978-0-595-74170-0 (cloth)
ISBN-10: 0-595-24337-1 (pbk)
ISBN-10: 0-595-74170-3 (cloth)

Printed in the United States of America

Contents

Foreword ix

Acknowledgements xv

PART I—DIAGNOSIS

Chapter 1   Learning The Anatomy 3

Chapter 2   Digital Rectal Examination (DRE): The Magic Finger 7

Chapter 3   PSA—What Is It and How Accurate 11

Chapter 4   PSA II—A Better Choice 15

Chapter 5   Ultrasound—Another Way of Looking 19

Chapter 6   Biopsy—How many core samples are enough? 21

Chapter 7   Negative Biopsy—It is really correct? 25

Chapter 8   Pelvic Lymph Node Dissection (PLND) 29

Chapter 9   Positron Emission Tomography—PET Scan 33

Chapter 10   Other Prostate Problems 35

               BPH—Benign Prostatic Hyperplasia 35

               Infections 38

               P I N 40

Chapter 11   Staging the Disease 43

Chapter 12   Gleason Scores 51

Chapter 13   Partin Tables 55

PART II—TREATMENT

Chapter 14   General Treatment Options 63

Chapter 15   Surgery 67

    Radical Surgery 68

    Cryosurgery—Temperature-Monitored Cryoablation of
the Prostate 73

    Microwave 75

    Robotic Surgery 78

Chapter 16   Radiation 79

    External Beam Radiation 80

    Conformal Proton Beam Radiation 81

    TomoTherapy 84

    Three Dimensional Conformal Radiation—(3D CRT) 84

    Intensity Modulated Radiation Therapy (IMRT) 87

    Brachytherapy—Seed Implantation 87

Chapter 17   Hormone Therapy 95

Chapter 18   Monoclonal Antibodies 101

Chapter 19   Holistic—The Herbal Approach 105

Chapter 20   Wait and Watch 113

Chapter 21   What Is The Right Treatment For You? 117

PART III—RECURRENCE CONSIDERATIONS

Chapter 22   Diagnosis 127

Chapter 23   Treatment Options 131

    Cryosurgery 132

    Hormone Treatment 132

    Chemotherapy 133

    Radiation 135

    Vaccine 135

Chapter 24 What To Do If The Cancer Returns 137

PART IV—CONCLUSION

Summary Remarks 141

PART V—REFERENCE MATERIAL

Websites 153

Organizations 157

The Partin Tables 161

Illustrations 165

Glossary 171

Foreword

Eight years ago I sat down and addressed the problem of how to get information out about prostate cancer and its treatments. Like most men, I found myself enmeshed in my career and with the usual concerns about family, friends, finances, and everyday living. Missing from my busy schedule was both awareness and interest in health problems.

Having spent many years in various pursuits, I considered myself reasonably intelligent and worldly. I shared with most American men a sense of self-assurance, which did not include the need for periodic physical examinations. In fact having spent over thirty years in association with the United States Air Force, both on Active Duty and in the Reserves, I was convinced of my good health and good fortune. Every so many years the Air Force would send me notes to secure a complete physical examination. I had to maintain my weight within certain parameters, which I was absolutely certain, would guaranty me immortality.

Ten years would elapse between my retiring from the United States Air Force Reserves and my next encounter with a "physical examination." In fact this fateful occurrence still would not have taken place were it not for the fact a good friend of mine as a result of taking a physical examination was determined to have colon cancer. With some considerable pressure from friendly health zealots around me, I finally consented to submit to a colonoscopy in order to determine whether I, too, would find myself confronted with intestinal cancer. I generally felt fine. Other then the usual minor aches and pains, which disappeared after a hot bathtub, I was not

predisposed to believe the examination was essential. Prior to the procedure, the physician who was to perform the procedure decided that since
it had been so long since my last comprehensive examination, a complete
blood work-up would make a lot of sense. To this day I firmly believe that
the good physician, who incidentally is a personal friend, felt that this
might be his only opportunity to ascertain whether I was still alive!

The blood test was something I had experienced before. I had nothing to
eat or drink from midnight of the previous night. The glee with which the
nurse drew the blood from the vein in the middle of my arm initially rein-
forced my reasons for avoiding physicians. Within a few days the results
were back. Within the overall analysis, everything was reasonable for a
man who was fifty-nine years of age with one glaring and major exception—my PSA level was 11.5! Little did I know then that this result would
set into motion a series of events which not only lead to the discovery of
the existence of prostate cancer, but also the mine field of options and
confusion pertaining to the treatment of the disease. Perhaps the single
most unsettling fact was that I felt fine and had no discernible perceptions
of anything awry in the body. The report, which contained all of the
results from the blood test, was in many ways a mixture of terms, some of
which I knew but the vast majority had no meaning to me whatsoever.
The only reality was to look at the laboratory's range of "normal values" in
order to determine where I stood. It was at this juncture concern for the
PSA level took on a deeper meaning since the "normal range" was between
0.0 and 4.0. I was not completely aware at this point just what this normal
PSA range signified. Not only was my reading considerably higher then
the normal range but I needed to now understand what PSA or "Prostate
Specific Antigen" signified.

Since that initial shock, I not only have learned a great deal about what
the PSA is, but also what it is not! Over the last few years, the medical
profession has reevaluated the significance of the PSA as an indicator of

potential problems. I have also come to realize that the PSA is not the whole picture and can in fact be very misleading.

The educational process I began when I was diagnosed continues to this very day. I have been fortunate to encounter honest physicians who were and continue to be supportive. Before my treatment they were willing to listen and discuss without betraying a sense of arrogant prejudice for one modality over another. However, it took me time, patience and confidence to arrive at what I could live with and accept as providing the best chance for a good prognosis and a quality of life that was more then merely a quantity of life. Each man will have to ultimately arrive at his own conclusions. The important thing to keep in mind is that you are the individual going through the illness. In the majority of diagnosed cases of prostate cancer you do have the time to educate yourself about the disease, treatment alternatives and prognosis. We are learning more and more about the causes and treatment of this disease all the time. Even the United States Government has gotten into the act when the U.S. Department of Veteran Affairs has determined if a man served in Vietnam and has developed prostate cancer, it is now considered to be a service connected disability.

Like the first book I wrote about prostate cancer, this book seeks to provide the start of your education into understanding prostate cancer and its treatments. I have attempted to update this new edition by discussing the latest developments in both diagnosis and treatment. Further, recognizing that prostate cancer can and often reoccurs, I have added a chapter on reoccurrence. New studies are constantly being discussed and published in leading medical journals. Included in this edition are the most recent studies. This new edition is not intended to be a biography of my experiences. To the extent I inject myself into the discussion, it is done only to aid in the explanation process. What you learn by reading this book will be important not only for yourself but also for those loved ones with whom you live and who care about you. Every day new information becomes available concerning prostate cancer treatments. The rest is up to the reader to enlarge the basis of their understanding, always keeping in mind that through knowledge you achieve comprehension and through comprehension ultimately the ability to make the right treatment decision for you! Whatever decision you determine is the right one for yourself must make you feel confident and comfortable.

STUART R. WOLK, Ph.D., JD
May 2007

CONSULTANTS IN UROLOGY, P.A.

MALCOLM SCHWARTZ, M.D.   BERNARD J. LEHRHOFF, M.D.
KENNETH S. RING, M.D.   MARK I. MILLER, M.D.

Diplomates American Board of Urology

Male Infertility   Adult and Pediatric Urology   Sexual Dysfunction

275 Orchard Street, Westfield, N.J. 07090 908-0654-5100   659 Kearny Avenue, Kearny, N.J. 07032 201-997-0640

318 Chestnut Street, Roselle Park, NJ. 07204 908-241-5268   743 Northfield Avenue, West Orange, N.J. 07032973-325-0091

Fax 908-654-8021

I have had the pleasure of reading A Man's Dilemma by Dr. Stuart Wolk.

This book, although written by the author as well as a patient is not a biography.

He has written a very concise treatise on prostate cancer, which is extremely informative and easy to understand for the lay person. It is very accurate in regard to the medical information depicted, and will assist any person who wishes to become more informed on the subject matter. Whether you be a patient or a family member, it will guide you through the diagnosis and treatment options available to you. I highly recommend this book to all.

Acknowledgements

This revision of the First Edition continues to be dedicated to every man and their families who will undergo the trauma of being told they have prostate cancer.

To the dedicated physicians who not only treated me but showed concern and patience with my attempts at humor, especially to Morton Marks MD, a friend and confidant I utilized as a virtual medical encyclopedia while making my treatment choices and has continued to this day to provide sound advice. To Bernard Lehrhoff MD, urologist, I discovered a rare find in a physician who has not only provided solid medical advice and support but has been willing to share his expertise in so many areas of this book. He not only read and helped in the editing of this manuscript but served to interpret many of the medical issues I have periodically raised. To Andrew Zablow MD, radiation oncologist, who read the manuscript and provided me with insight and encouragement. To Mark Waxman MD, who with his quiet manner and willingness to put up with my questions ultimately became the catalyst for this book.

To Alan Shoemaker, a friend for all seasons who became scared while reading the manuscript and undertook to edit it with care and concern and to this very day has found time to always be there for me.

To my wife Priscilla who, although she has endured her own traumatic medical problems, has sustained me throughout the ordeal and continues to provide support when my spirits lag.

PART I

DIAGNOSIS

Chapter 1

Learning The Anatomy

Every man at some point in his life undergoes a thorough examination that includes the probing of his rectum by his physician. In spite of my enduring this indignity, I candidly have to admit I was never certain just exactly what the physician was looking for. In the process of my coming to grips with my diagnosis of prostate cancer I suddenly realized that to understand fully the significance of this Digital Rectal Examination (DRE for short), I needed to know something about the prostate gland itself. It was somewhat of an embarrassment to me to realize that I knew so little about the location, purpose, and function of this walnut shaped gland. This ignorance of the various aspects of one's body illustrates not only a failure of the educational processes, but also explains why so many individuals fail to seek medical treatment before serious symptoms occur. Although I had rectal examinations during my association with the United States Air Force, I never gave much attention to the significance of the process. As is the case with most men, I found the examination to be both psychologically and physically uncomfortable and was only too happy when it was over. My embarrassment was further magnified when I started to study my anatomy. I was basically ignorant of how my reproductive system functioned. Women, unlike men, have a keen awareness of their bodily functions and the particular functionality of all aspects of their reproductive system; from fallopian tubes to ovaries, cervix to uterus, women from puberty onward have a monthly reminder of their "system." Additionally, once through puberty, most women visit a gynecologist periodically. Pap smears and breast examinations are constantly touted in the media as mechanisms for preventing and catching diseases before they cause serious harm. Conversely, men are told very little about their reproductive process other than being aware from youth onward that they possess a penis and testicles. Ask most men what the seminal vesicles or the vas deferens are, and they will look at you as though you are describing a foreign war scene. Throw in cowpers glands and more esoteric names such as verumontanum, and ischiopubic ramus, and you may get a left hook to the jaw. Many well-educated men I know will even talk about the "prostrate" when they mean the "prostate." Even men who may have some familiarity with the various aspects of their anatomy do not seem to know what role these different structures play in the reproductive process. Why this ignorance persists is a puzzle. Perhaps part of the answer may lie in the fact that men do not have the monthly cycle women endure. The very role women play in bearing children has created the greater awareness.

There is another aspect to the ignorance men have about their body. Until very recently, the general media and medical advertisements have forgotten that there are both men and women in the human race. All medical advertising until very recently appears to have been directed solely at women. This has only changed with men such as General Schwartzkopf, Senator Dole, New York City's Mayor and New York Yankees Manager Joe Torre coming forward announcing that they had prostate cancer. Followed by the marketing of Viagra, Levitra and Cialis, it would appear that only small aspects of potential male problems have been illuminated. Erectile Dysfunction has become the major focus of advertising to men as though this were a new problem and now okay to discuss in mixed company!

I became aware of my own lack of comprehension and quickly decided that I not only needed a refresher in Biology 101, but also to gain a greater understanding of the interrelationship between all of the essential aspects of the male reproductive system. If I were to make an intelligent decision pertaining to my treatment, I had better learn what the risks to each of the various functions of the system would be if surgery, radiation, or some other form of the treatment were undertaken. I was not interested in becoming a urologist, but I certainly should have as comparable a knowledge of "me" as women do of themselves. What surprised me in my research was how easy it was to find definitions that even the layman could understand. Dictionaries were a good jumping off point, and a basic college biology book with a diagram of the human reproductive system provided further data. As I proceeded to investigate further, my own personal need was to delve beyond the fundamentals and to become more knowledgeable. I finally settled on a medical textbook that had some wonderful full color charts on what was functioning inside of me. What became critical to my investigation was where some of these functions were located in relationship to the prostate gland.

Basically, I knew that the prostate gland definition is by definition a male sex gland. Together with the testicles and the seminal vesicles, it is part of the process by which sperm cells are ultimately ejaculated. In simple terms: together with the seminal vesicles, the prostate gland aids in supplying the fluid in which the sperm travel to be ejaculated through the urethra. There are many separate functions being performed in order for the sperm to go from the testicles to the ultimate ejaculation. Some of the ancillary anatomy is located outside of the prostate gland itself, and some is involved within the prostate through various ducts. This I learned provides concern to the patient and the physician alike. If a malignancy exists, it can and often spreads beyond the prostate gland itself into the surrounding tissue such as the seminal vesicles. The actual physical location of the prostate is below the bladder. I discovered that the prostate completely surrounds the urethra, the tube through which both urine and semen travel. The fact that the prostate surrounds the urethra can cause all types of problems for men, not only those associated with cancer. It also appears that as men age there is a general enlargement of the gland that can cause pressure on the urethra, making it difficult to urinate. As I was to find out later, urologists love to measure the "flow rate" of urinating in order to ascertain whether there are problems with the urethra as a result of this enlargement. Candidly, I must admit, prior to my experience with prostate cancer, I never thought much about my prostate-urinary functioning, just so long as everything appeared to be "working!" In spite of numerous medical examinations throughout my military career, no physician ever explained the nuances of the male reproductive system. Nor were there discussions concerning the interrelationships between the component parts. This was all to change, and I suspect that for the rest of my life, I shall be conscious of the workings of my plumbing!

Chapter 2

Digital Rectal Examination (DRE): The Magic Finger

Human anatomy can be extremely interesting when it is your own! The location of the rectum, lying immediately behind the bladder, prostate gland and seminal vesicles, allows the physician to feel the gland through the rectal wall by inserting a finger up the rectum. The well-trained physician will feel irregular shapes or lumps and also hardness in some cases, which may give rise to suspicions concerning the health of the gland. It is by no means a conclusive test and must be viewed together with the results of the PSA test and other symptoms. In other words, to the physician the gland may feel normal, but you may still have disease.

The examination itself is painless … and embarrassing for most men. You must bend over the examining table, drop your pants and underwear, and be "probed!" It provides a parallel to what women must encounter when examined vaginally by a gynecologist. Since the onset of the diagnosis of my prostate cancer, I have stopped being critical of comments made by female friends complaining about the "indignity of medical examinations." Nonetheless, it is a small price to pay if the probing ultimately leads to discovery of any problem and its treatment. After all, dignity is in the mind of the individual and some things in life must fall under the heading of having to "grin and bear it." By inserting a finger into the rectum, the physician can feel both sides of the prostate. My research soon clarified exactly what the physician was seeking when a finger is placed in the rectum. The gland should not have any hard or calcified areas. Any nodes or extensions from the smooth surface of the gland may indicate a problem. Through the digital examination, the physician can also get an idea of the size of the gland and determine in a preliminary manner whether the gland is enlarged. Enlargement does not necessarily indicate a malignancy, but may give evidence of other disorders such as BPH, a condition I will discuss later on in the book which can prevent you from urinating properly among other symptoms. It was discomforting to be told by my physician that an enlarged prostate is also common as "you age!"

If the digital examination feels "normal," to the physician there still may be a problem with the prostate. Further blood tests given in a routine fashion will measure the PSA, as a follow up to the digital examination will provide a better idea of the condition of the gland. Most early diagnosis of prostate cancer does not get discovered through the use of the digital examination alone. If the physician feels any irregularity on either side of the prostate, further tests will need to be undertaken. As most physicians have told me during my treatment the best "educated finger" is not a substitute for follow up tests. This is one of the areas of great concern. At what point do you as a patient feel confident? You cannot rely on the DRE alone even if the physician tells you they have felt no abnormalities. I reviewed all of my prior Air Force physicals, copies of which I secured upon retirement. Each physical examination had a notation that a digital rectal examination had been performed. I cannot help but wonder how long the cancer was growing in my prostate and whether it existed at the time when any of the Air Force examinations were performed?

Since the end of my treatment, every visit to the urologist has included not only a PSA test but also a DRE to ascertain if the physician can feel any changes to the prostate. My prostate not having been removed, the DRE can provide an initial indication of reoccurrence or enlargement due to other causes. Fortunately, my prostate has continued to be extremely small and showing no signs of abnormal changes.

Chapter 3

PSA—What Is It and How Accurate

The follow up test to the DRE is a blood test to determine your PSA.PSA stands for "prostate specific antigen". Until the late 1980's, this test did not exist. Prior to 1980, physicians had to rely on the digital rectal examination and whatever symptoms the patient indicated. The ensuing results were not good. Within my own family and circle of friends, prostate cancer was viewed as a disease of the older male with all of the other urinary infirmities that seemed associated with the male aging process. I recall that my father-in-law had his prostate removed (a prostatectomy) due to a serious enlargement and difficulty with urination. In his hospital ward, there were eight other men who also had undergone the same procedure. All of them appeared to be between their late sixties and early seventies. With the development of the PSA test, early diagnosis theoretically became more accurate. This can be illustrated by the increase in both the numbers of younger men discovered with the disease, and the numbers at earlier stages. The obvious conclusion to be drawn is that prostate cancer and other prostate problems are not confined to the elderly, but are to be found in younger men as well.

Attempting to define meanings of terms and the significance of tests is a major problem for men diagnosed with prostate cancer. The physician tells you that a blood test is needed in order to measure your PSA. Unfortunately that information doesn't tell you much. What exactly is PSA? I soon found out that PSA is a protein produced by the prostate and is found in extremely small amounts in the blood stream. When cancer, injury, disease or inflammation has affected the gland the level of PSA in the bloodstream tends to rise. The PSA level can also rise when the gland becomes enlarged. It is part of the semen and is even in the urine. It is a normal part of the process of the gland. It is this "overflow" into the blood stream that gives rise to suspicions that something may be wrong in the gland. There is another factor however, if a man is on medication, the level of PSA may be giving the physician a false reading. This is especially true if the individual is under some form of hormone therapy, since the prostate is "hormone sensitive."

In recent years there has been a growing controversy about the effectiveness of the PSA test and whether it is an indicator of cancer. Some physicians have even argued the test does not provide consistent proof of the presence of prostate cancer to be worth while. Recently the United States Department of Defense entered into this debate and let it be known that the PSA test was not a standard blood test given to men over fifty or African-American servicemen over forty. This ongoing debate concerning the value of the PSA test is unsettling to say the least. In the late 1980's I was given a "retirement physical examination by the Air Force. As a senior ranking officer, the treatment I received was thorough. I recall that the examining physician asked me if I wanted a new test to see if I had prostate cancer. I asked about the test and was informed that it was a blood test, but "it is not totally proven, and besides your are still rather young to have prostate cancer!" "I took the test anyway and didn't get the results for three months. It was "on the high side," so I was told.

As you confront these facts you must be prepared to understand that standing alone the PSA test may be inconclusive. Do these mean that you should ignore the PSA results if they appear to be higher then the normal range? As important if the PSA comes back within normal ranges does that mean that you do not have prostate cancer? In spite of these debates, until a better diagnostic method becomes available, the PSA test is still the simplest and cheapest method to detect possible changes in the prostate caused by cancer or other disorders. Recognize that several PSA tests may be needed in order to ascertain whether a problem exists with the prostate. This is one of the more frustrating aspects of dealing with prostate cancer. A single PSA test may not be sufficient. Nine months before I was diagnosed with prostate cancer I had a very elevated PSA of 11.5. My next PSA test three months later was 0.72. Five months thereafter I had a PSA of 13.5! By June of the same year utilizing a newer PSA test, the level had risen to 16.5.

What is not altogether clear is what the "normal" level of PSA is when a test is taken. Of course, the test is taken by extracting a blood sample, so be prepared to be "stuck" again! A high level of PSA may create suspicions, but it does not guarantee that you have cancer. Age and other conditions can raise the PSA beyond the so-called normal range. One of the distinct problems with the human body is that what is "normal" may be hard to define. Absent any other evidence of disease except an elevated PSA, a series of tests may be a good idea to see if there are changes in the level from test to test. Remember that the PSA level is measured in "nanograms per milliliter," which, if I remember my college science courses, is an extremely small amount of substance.

Increases in the PSA level appearing in three or four tests over a six month period may give some indication that cancer is present, especially if the rate of increase is significant. Keep in mind those other problems indicated above which may cause the PSA level to become elevated, one of the most common being a condition called, "prostititus." As I personally progressed through several PSA tests I was becoming increasingly aware of friends and acquaintances that had PSA levels within the normal range only to find out as the result of biopsies that prostate cancer was present. In fact in one situation a friend with a PSA level of 3.72 had several core samples of his biopsy indicate prostate cancer. Some of these individuals also discovered that when the pathologist had completed their investigations, the Gleason Scores measuring the aggressiveness of the cancer indicated fairly active cancers. Recent studies reported in the New England Journal of Medicine in July 2004 seem to indicate that the significance of the PSA may be related more to the rate of increase prior to diagnosis of prostate cancer than to the actual number itself. This does not mean however that higher numbers are not significant.

If the digital examination does not disclose any suspicious abnormalities, there is still no guarantee that prostate cancer is not present. In many ways this is part of the problem in the diagnosis of prostate cancer. Absent clear clinical evidence of some prostate problem, cancer can exist without an elevated PSA. The obvious "chicken or the egg" question immediately rears its head. If all of these doubts exist should I even bother with the PSA test? The answer has to be "yes!" With all of the uncertainty men must start at some point to begin the process of investigating the possibilities of existence of prostate cancer. It is not altogether clear at what age the PSA test needs to be given. Unsettling stories of men in their thirties with prostate cancer has to make one wonder whether the guidelines of 50 years of age for Caucasian men and 40 years of age for African men may not be safe absolutes. If the test is recommended to be given at younger ages will men bother with taking the test? Youth tends to have a sense of immortality that creates difficulties convincing them to accept the potential of prostate cancer at such young years.

Chapter 4

PSA II—A Better Choice

A newer PSA test has recently been developed, known as "PSA II." These tests look for "Free PSA" in the blood. Without going into the technical differences, the "Free PSA" is measured and results in a percentage. The higher the percentage of "Free PSA," the lesser the probability of prostate cancer. Most testing laboratories consider that if the percentage of "Free PSA" is 25% or greater, the man is within normal ranges. Watch that word "probability." The PSA and "Free PSA" are merely tools and do not definitively prove the existence of cancer in the gland.

As I indicated before I had a PSA test given to me by an Air Force physician in the early days of the test. The test had to be sent out by the Air Force Hospital since these tests were new and not generally given. When the test result came back it was "on the high side" which ultimately translated to 8.0. In those years no one seemed to understand what was a "normal" level and no one at that time indicated anything to me about the significance of the test. I also had a digital rectal examination at that time, which, according to the physician was "normal." Did that indicate I had cancer ten years before it was finally diagnosed? Although it was unlikely because the cancer can be very slow growing, the possibility does exist. These factors lead one to the obvious conclusion that the digital rectal examination and the PSA test must be undertaken frequently and at least every year after the age of 50. If you are an African-American male or an individual with a history of prostate or breast cancer in your immediate family, then starting these tests at an earlier age would appear to be statistically sound.

There is one area of concern whether we are talking about the PSA or the PSA II test, namely, how accurate are they? In my case, after the initial test and before I took the PSA II, I had a second PSA taken ninety days later. This test through the same physician came back "0.72." This provided the first lesson in taking command of my own future treatment. This second test also illustrates the conscious and subconscious desire to hope for the best and not press the issue of the accuracy of results. Although I doubted the ability of the PSA to drop so much, I was willing to accept the answer that I may have had an infection that would have accounted for the initial elevated PSA. I wanted to hear that everything was fine and that I did not have cancer. As I will discuss later, I did have a biopsy after the initial PSA reading. This biopsy came back—negative! Therefore, the two tests taken together indicated that prostate-wise I appeared to be in fine health. In retrospect, I should have had a retest of the second PSA reading, or at least a PSA II test, to confirm the apparent miraculous drop in the PSA score. Some individuals will argue that their insurance will not cover two tests so close together. The answer to that concern in this environment of "health by the bottom line," is that your life must take precedence over what the Insurance Company will allow.

The failure to take the retest of the PSA cost me six months time before the ultimate discovery of my cancer. What this delay will mean in my long-term prognosis is clearly too early to know. The only advantage I have is that prostate cancer tends to be a slow growing disease. There are no easy answers especially when you have no symptoms. If I were to look back, the rate of increase of my PSA would indicate some dire long term potential for reoccurrence. This may still be the long-term result over the next five years or so. To date, however, my PSA has settled down to an acceptable 0.3 except for the very last test where the result came back at 0.21 In light of my prior experience with a drop in my PSA level prior to my original diagnosis of prostate cancer, I should question why this drop of one-third of the PSA level. However, I am seven and one-half years from my original diagnosis and seven plus years from my last treatment for the disease. All of the indications are presently good and the drop in the PSA level is not statistically out of line with the past two years of tests.

The University of Texas Health Science Center in San Antonio, Texas has studied a small select group of men who did not test positive for prostate cancer. Their study seemed to indicate that if a man was fat the PSA tended to be lower. Obviously if you are relying on the PSA result alone, this can be misleading to the physician and patient alike. This study is even more significant when it has been shown in other research that prostate cancer is more aggressive in over-weight men.

If the University of Texas study were not enough, I am troubled further by a recent publication I encountered aimed at senior citizens, which indicated that if a man has no symptoms and is over 70 years of age, an annual PSA is not needed. I find this recommendation from a physician to be extremely troubling. Like me, many men will evince no symptoms and have no discomfort. Seventy years of age is not what it was fifty years past. Most seventy-year-old men in the Western Industrial World are still vibrant and can look forward to years of productivity. Although the PSA test may not be the entire answer, a needle prick and a little blood taking every year is a small price to pay for knowledge!

Chapter 5

Ultrasound—Another Way
of Looking

As I was soon to find out, prostate cancer and prostate disorders in general have a unique way of humbling most men. Not only do you submit to the digital rectal examination, but also if the PSA is high, and the DRE does not seem to provide the physician with a sense that there is some abnormality, an ultrasound may be taken to determine if there is a clear evidence of disease. Having stated the ultrasound test in a matter of fact manner, it may be more graphic to provide its full name: "transrectal ultrasound," or "TRUS" for short. While this procedure is not painful in most cases, like most prostate examination procedures, it is uncomfortable. The ultrasound device is inserted in the rectum in order to secure a picture of the prostate, computerized, and reduced to a printable file representation or projected on a monitor. Needless to say, this marvel of modern diagnostic instrumentation is somewhat larger then the physician's "educated finger!"

It is remarkable how at this stage in my mid-life I have been reduced so many times to assuming the fetal position in order to be probed and examined. I truly believe that my prostate has been palpated (felt) and photographed more than any other portion of my anatomy. There is comfort nonetheless in knowing that the physician's educated finger can be important in providing an indication of the status of the gland. My physician has recently informed me that the size of my gland is probably in the range of 5-10cc. Prior to treatment, as I will discuss more fully later in the book, the gland was an extremely large (65.3cc).

Once again, it must be understood that ultrasound is not a definitive diagnostic answer to elevated PSA levels or even uncertain digital examinations. In the earliest stages of prostate cancer, the ultrasound may not show any evidence of the presence of cancer. Ultrasound can, however, indicate the presence of other problems such as retention of urine in the bladder. This condition can give rise to infections. Perhaps this is one of the most troubling aspects of prostate cancer. Modern medicine informs men and women to seek periodic examinations for suspected disorders. Yet, even with the most sophisticated diagnostic equipment and tests, there is absolutely no guarantee that they will definitively establish the existence or nonexistence of a disease. It is because of these realities that when either the PSA is high or the physician believes there may be evidence of a problem resulting from the digital rectal examination, the next step may need to be undertaken: a biopsy. Alternatively, additional PSA tests could be taken over a period of time. There is a certain comfort in resolving a problem rather then my playing the role of ostrich. Clearly, the very thought of a biopsy sends chills down the spine of most people. The method of doing the biopsy, once explained to many men, also creates some nervousness. Nonetheless, from my perspective, I find that living with uncertainty, even over a relatively short time frame, is not acceptable.

Chapter 6

Biopsy—How many core samples are enough?

Where does this lead someone if the DRE, PSA and ultrasound are not conclusive? The next obvious step has got to be the invasive "biopsy!" The very word—"biopsy," always seems to conjure up images from some Boris Karloff movie. Ignorance of the manner in which the procedure is performed also creates levels of anxiety that most men would prefer to do without. In December 1997 when I had been informed that my PSA level was 11.5, the need to perform a biopsy became more apparent when the digital examination indicated an enlarged gland with one side presenting evidence of thickening. The next step was to find a competent urologist to perform the biopsy. As a typical male, I did not know any urologist. I had no prior urinary problems that would have necessitated seeking one out. My first instinct was to ask a close family friend who was associated with a major New York City University medical center. I was within commuting distance of New York, and having an office within Manhattan initially made the use of a New York City facility appealing. However, if there were to be additional procedures required, convenience to home had to be a consideration as well. Although I grew up in New York City and must admit to a certain prejudice about "everything New York," I have learned to accept the fact that there are equally competent professionals West of the Hudson River. I had tremendous faith in the gastroenterologist, who had discovered the PSA level, so I felt at ease asking him for a referral. As luck would have it, he spoke very highly of a urologist associated with him in the same local hospital located in of all places New Jersey and convenient to my home.

It is important to note that selecting the right physician is critical. Not only must you have confidence in the capabilities of the individual, but the physician must also have a compatible personality. The skill of the physician is critical in any treatment, yet, in potentially life threatening diseases, the need to have a rapport with the treating physician is just as important. Keep in mind that it is your health and your concerns that are at stake. I find it difficult to deal with a physician who has no time for a little TLC (tender loving care). Like chicken soup, it may not help, but it sure as heck can't hurt! If you do not know a urologist, some networking with friends and associates quite often turns up names and impressions. Even with a recommendation, once you make an appointment do not be afraid to ask the physician the appropriate questions, such as: how long has the physician been in practice; where did he or she train; and with what hospitals is he or she affiliated.

My initial biopsy in December 1997 was performed in the office of the urologist. I have considered myself as an individual who has been around the world and can usually refrain from becoming neither embarrassed nor uneasy. The procedure, however, had an unnerving effect. It was not the discomfort of lying on my side with my knees up to my chest. It was not the insertion of the biopsy probe with the transrectal ultrasound. Rather, it was the presence of an attractive technician along with the urologist that did me in! The biopsy is conducted without any anesthesia. Although I was somewhat tense, not knowing what to expect, I did not feel any pain when the biopsy was conducted. The only sensation was a feeling of pressure when the biopsy needle took the sample and the "popping" sound when the biopsy needle deployed. When the biopsy was concluded, I was given some antibiotic pills to take for several days and informed about a potential for two other side effects:—the possibility of blood in the urine, and the second was blood in the ejaculation. All in all, although unpleasant, I left the urologist's office in about the same condition as I had arrived, and went directly to work.

When I received the results of the biopsy approximately one week later, I discovered that there were six samples that had been taken during the procedure. Three were removed from each side of the gland. In the course of my subsequent research, I learned that the size of the gland has a major bearing on the number of samples taken during the biopsy procedure. This is especially true if the transrectal ultrasound has not indicated the presence of the cancer. If the urologist follows a standard sample-taking approach as where to take the samples, if the prostate gland is enlarged (very common in older men) a small number of biopsy samples may miss the malignant cells, especially if they are in small random clusters within the gland.

As the future would illustrate, in November 1998, my second biopsy of eight samples came back with two samples being positive. This indicated that less than 5% of the gross tissue was malignant. Just how the pathologist calculates the percentage of malignant cells is not clear. What I subsequently discovered was that the percentage of the gross samples that are malignant can be a significant factor in the prognosis of the patient. The additional core samples that were taken managed to hit the cancer. If eight samples been taken in December 1997, would they have discovered the cancer? No one will ever be able to answer that question. What is important is that questions need to be asked of the urologist when a biopsy is to be performed. Specifically, what is the size of the gland? How many samples do you intend to take? If the gland appears to be over 40cc, then determine whether more samples are needed, especially if no tumor is visible or palpable. A close friend of mine with a large gland had a total of ten samples taken: five on either side of the gland. When I questioned him as to why this large number of biopsy samples he had no answer. I suspect it the number of samples must have had something to do with the size of his prostate. Since I wrote the first edition of this book I have spoken to many men who have had their prostate glands biopsied. The number of core samples taken has ranged from four to twelve with no reasonable explanation given to them as to why so many were taken.

I marvel at how I underwent the biopsy procedure with virtually no questions being asked of the urologist. For all of my subsequent investigation, at one of the most critical points in my diagnosis, I was still leaving everything up to the physician. I believe most men suffer from the feeling that "real men do not question or complain." Older men who have been in the military almost seem to salute smartly and accept whatever comes their way.

Chapter 7

Negative Biopsy—It is really correct?

One week after the initial December 1997 biopsy, the results came back—negative. All six core samples showed no evidence of cancer. The general view of the urologist was that there was either an infection of the prostate or some inflammation. In any event, my relief was noticeable and comforting. I just wanted to forget about the prostate and that I had undergone the anxiety and worry that had accompanied the entire two months.

Perhaps my initial experience with the examination process illustrates the importance of not becoming overly confident with results. Prostate cancer is a strange disease. You can have it, be examined, and still appear to be free of the disease. Constant vigilance is the watchword with this malignancy. Even with a negative report, you need to maintain a schedule of periodic examinations, especially if you are over 50 years of age, or younger if an African—American. The tendency to feel a sense of relief with a negative biopsy can lull you into false security. I returned to the urologist within three months of the biopsy finding and had another digital examination, along with a new temperature probe and a new PSA. In effect, I was following up and doing the "right thing." The results were encouraging. The digital and temperature examination appeared normal. The PSA came back 0.72. The sudden drop from a PSA level of 11.5 to 0.72 raised questions in my mind, but with all other factors seeming to be in place, who was I to question further? As the saying goes, "why trouble, trouble?" Even the examining physician seemed to take comfort in the drop, indicating that everything else appeared to be normal and writing off the initial high PSA to perhaps an infection or irritation.

The lesson to be learned is that the tendency for most people to resort to the ostrich approach to matters pertaining to their bodies can result in disaster. Fortunately, prostate cancer is generally slow growing and provides some forgiveness for general stupidity. In retrospect, I should have insisted upon a second PSA to validate or invalidate this sudden decline in my PSA. Once again, the important lesson to be understood is that your health is ultimately within your own hands. What does not make sense needs to be examined further, even if the physician does not see the purpose behind your concerns. As subsequent events indicated, my urologist might have thought me crazy, but he is not the type of person who would have obstructed my desire for a re-testing. The fault lay at my feet. Even if your physician does not believe there is a necessity of a re-examination, remember that it is your body! If the insurance carrier does not reimburse you for the re-test, remember that it is your body! If your spouse or significant other gives you a funny look and believes you have become a hypochondriac, remember that it is your body! I am presently attempting to convince a very good friend, age 65, whose PSA has reached 19.1 that in spite of three negative biopsies over the past five years, he needs to pre-server and if necessary seek a second or third opinion.

After the results of my second biopsy, I was stunned! Deep down I have to admit that at some level I understood how unlikely my initial feeling that this second biopsy was going to be normal. When I reflected on the increasing PSA level and a PSA II test I took on my own which indicated a

16.5, I knew that a second biopsy would not be good. I asked the urologist about how common it is to have a negative biopsy and to discover the cancer at some subsequent point in time. The answer was that it is not uncommon, even with elevated PSA levels. The answer to the next query became more chilling. When would the urologist have wanted to see me again if the second biopsy had been negative? Next year! Just how significant would waiting another year have been to the long-term prognosis? No one can answer that question. The more the disease is studied the more there is evidence that prostate cancer may fall into two categories, with one being more aggressive than the other. If you are fortunate to have a less aggressive form then the delay in diagnosis may not have any real significance. On the other hand, if you have the more aggressive form, there is some evidence that even early diagnosis may not be necessarily effective since the treatment in such cases may not necessarily alter the ultimate progression of the disease. The push is now on to be able to differentiate between the two forms and determine what is the best approach to treatment.

The question I have been asked over the last few years from clients and friends is one that continues to raise issues within the medical community. At what age should a man "stop" being screened for prostate cancer? Assuming that a large percentage of prostate cancers are slow growing, should a man over the age of 75 or 80 continue to have his PSA measured or undergo a DRE? In December 2003, a study conducted by the Cancer Institute of New Jersey confronted this problem and questioned not only the effectiveness of the PSA test itself but also whether it made any sense to continue testing into old age. Clearly from a statistical perspective, the odds of a man over the age of 75 dying from newly discovered early stage prostate cancer would seem to be remote. The problem, however, is that as a generalization people are living not only longer, but also more active, productive lives. Living into the late eighties or even into the nineties is no longer an oddity. Perhaps the more interesting issue would be if prostate cancer is discovered in a man 75 or 80 years of age, what treatment should they undergo … if any?

Chapter 8

Pelvic Lymph Node Dissection (PLND)

I began to recognize that everything I was doing was like a puzzle with various pieces being put into place. When the biopsy comes back indicating the presence of cancer what further tests are needed? Will additional tests give any better answers as to the extent of the disease? Here again, there is considerable debate as to what tests should be undertaken once prostate cancer has been diagnosed. Bone scans, which require the injecting of a small radioactive material, are widely utilized to test for spread to the bones, a usual location for metastases. Are these bone scans necessary? Some research indicates that patients whose cancer was discovered by high PSA levels followed by a positive biopsy may not need a bone scan, especially if the PSA level was below 20.

MRI, magnetic resonance imaging, is also utilized to detect spread of the cancer. Some physicians feel that if the Gleason score is 6 or under and the stage of the disease appears early, a MRI may not be warranted. This attitude appears more prevalent when the patient has opted for surgery, his Gleason Score is 6 or below, and he is in the early stage of the disease. The Gleason Score system, which attempts to define the relative aggressiveness of the cancer, will be discussed later on in the book. If the patient under-goes a radical prostatectomy, the surgeon will undoubtedly remove the lymph nodes located in the pelvic region in order to have a pathologist examine them. However, after considerable research and questioning I ascertained that not all of the surgical procedures allow for the removal of the lymph node. In those situations, or when a decision is made not to undergo surgery, issues arise as to whether to perform a pelvic lymph node dissection, PLND, as a separate procedure from whatever other treatment you may have decided to undertake.

The PLND is performed by an incision in the abdomen utilizing a device called a laparoscope. If this procedure is performed as a separate operation, it is far less invasive than the prostatectomy. Nonetheless, it is surgery, and although it can determine whether there is lymph involvement, whether it is necessary is still a question. The purpose of this diagnostic test must be viewed in the light of how the results will change the treatment for the dis-ease. In some ways, whether to have a PLND is a Catch-22. The risk of spread to the lymph node is statistically less with low Gleason scores, early stages, and low PSA levels. On the other hand, the PLND will indicate definitively whether there is lymph involvement. Although I cannot speak for other prostate cancer patients, I opted not to have the procedure because my test results did not seem to warrant undergoing this form of surgery. Candidly, my concern upon being informed I had prostate cancer was basic; will I ever be able to have sexual relations again; will I become incontinent? The thought of any form of surgical procedure was still in the distant future. Time will tell whether my decision was correct.

At some point in time in the treatment of any disease, determinations must be made as to where to draw the line and when to proceed with the rest of your life. Like everything else concerning prostate cancer, even assuming you decided to undergo a PLND, has this procedure helped you to decide the proper follow on treatment? Will the results alter the treatment you would prefer in any case?

Chapter 9

Positron Emission Tomography—PET Scan

The interesting situation you will encounter in your early confusion relating to diagnosing your condition is that new tests come out all the time. No sooner did I believe that I understood the next step in the diagnosis of my condition, then a new test was being discussed. Medicine is constantly developing new techniques for the diagnosis of disease. One of the newer diagnostic technologies is Positron Emission Tomography. (PET) has enabled physicians to better see into the human body through the use of metabolic markers. This is accomplished through a simple injection of any number of substances called markers that are linked to a specific chemical, attracted to only specific types of cells in the body. The ultimate image is three-dimensional and unlike other forms of scanning a more accurate diagnosis of the tumor can be determined to ascertain whether it is malignant or benign. The problem with this diagnostic procedure is not every hospital possesses the capability to perform it and the costs are on the high side.

The advantage of a PET Scan is that it can provide earlier diagnosis then other forms of diagnostic tests although it has not yet been proven extremely effective for early stage prostate cancer. Even after the discovery and treatment of the cancer, it can detect whether the cancer has returned and how extensive it is even if the patient has not become aware of the reoccurrence of the disease. If you are concerned about too many invasive procedures, this single pass test is relatively short in duration and of little if any discomfort. Relatively few hospitals possess the equipment, although at last investigation I was surprised at how many had managed to secure the capability. In large urban settings you are likely to find a major medical facility that has the equipment as well as the staff trained in its use.

A PET Scan is expensive, and is a test not reimbursed by many insurance companies. Since it is not altogether clear that it would alter treatment options, the dispute still continues whether to seek to undergo the procedure.

Chapter 10

Other Prostate Problems

BPH—Benign Prostatic Hyperplasia

It is remarkable how many disorders a man can develop involving his prostate. Ignorance may be bliss, but the more knowledge you possess can be overwhelming. I no sooner had discovered that I had prostate cancer, when I also found out I had this additional disorder—BPH. BPH (Benign Prostatic Hyperplasia) is not a malignant condition but it can present symptoms that are similar to prostate cancer. BPH can also have a major impact on the type of treatment you ultimately receive for the disease. The two disorders are such that if you have one you may or may not have the other. From what I have discovered, having BPH does not have anything to do with your risk of developing prostate cancer. However, BPH can mask the existence of prostate cancer, or make the cancer more difficult to detect. As with its more sinister cousin, BPH can also exist without any symptoms whatsoever. This was the situation I encountered. I had no idea that I had BPH. I had none of the usual problems common with this disorder. I had no problem urinating. I had no need to get up during the night with a sense of urgency to urinate. I had no perceptible reduction in the strength of the urine stream, nor starting and stopping urinating. In other words, I was a typical male, happy and slightly overweight. The lesson again is brought into focus that periodic examinations are absolutely essential to detect problems even before you are aware of their existence. So what is BPH and why did I even have to be concerned with its existence?

BPH by itself can cause an elevated PSA and needs to be understood since you can have both BPH and prostate cancer. Changes in the cellular structure of the prostate and results in an enlargement of the prostate cause BPH. If the prostate is often described as being "walnut size," BPH can cause it to enlarge beyond that of a large apricot and often results in difficulty in either urinating or in weakening the urine stream. This difficulty in urinating, referred to as "storage symptom," can lead to pain. More importantly, it can lead to infection in the bladder and kidneys, referred to as "voiding symptom." This can result in a constant urge to urinate, create difficulty in sleeping, and may even result in the need for protective undergarments. On the other hand, some individuals may never experience these problems and still have the disorder. While BPH usually is a symptom found in older men, it can occur at any age.

My prostate gland had enlarged to more than 65.3cc, a nice sized plum, with no apparent symptoms whatsoever. Nonetheless, BPH is far more common than prostate cancer and is the most common disorder in men with prostate problems. It is estimated that 80% of all prostate problems in men are BPH related. Although there is a tendency for the problem of BPH to worsen as time goes on, most men will not seek out treatment until there is difficulty or inability to urinate, burning urination, pain in urination, or bladder retention develop. The simple fact of life is that with all men, the prostate will continue to enlarge with age. At some point, you will probably find the need for some form of medical intervention. Medications such a Cardura are usually given to alleviate the symptoms and help to shrink the gland. Flomax, Detrol and similar newer medications may be given to regulate urine flow if urination becomes difficult or too frequent. The risk of infection along with the lessening of the bladder's ability to empty can also be the process of aging along with the gradual weakening of all of the muscles of the body. This does not mean that you have to go shopping for a final resting-place, just recognize you are no longer twenty years old! Tragically, some men believe that their life has ended once they have been diagnosed with either BPH or Prostate Cancer.

What is interesting is that the treatment for BPH can be very similar to those utilized for prostate cancer. Hormones can be used to attempt to shrink the gland. This was the situation I faced, since the size of my prostate was too big to allow for the treatment procedure I had selected known as seed implantation or brachytherapy. More often then not, a surgical procedure may be needed to remove some of the excess prostate tissue caused by the BPH condition. Called a "TURP," or "transurethral resection of the prostate." This is a fancy medical name for what is essentially the shaving down of the gland. The procedure is undertaken by inserting an instrument into the penis through the urethra. Passing through the urethra, some of the prostate tissue surrounding the urethra is removed. In scraping away the tissue, pressure is relieved and normal urination takes place again in most cases. Some physicians had informed me that once a person had a TURP certain prostate cancer treatments were no longer available. I have found such contradictory positions on this matter that frankly I am not certain urologist know the answer!

Concerned about the effect of all of the procedures and treatments I went through after I was diagnosed with prostate cancer, my urologist initially believed that my BPH condition and the resultant further swelling of the prostate might be causing retention of urine in my bladder. He suggested a TURP. Fortunately, after several sonograms of the bladder indicated no retention of urine, it was decided not to undertake this procedure. Whatever side effects I may have been experiencing from my treatment, I would be able to avoid any further invasive procedures. My urologist's initial invitation to have the TURP was avoided, much to my delight.

Being the typical male coward, the main reason I wanted to bypass the TURP was the usual necessity for a catheter to be inserted in the penis up to the bladder for a few days while recuperating from the procedure. While some individuals do not mind the presence of a catheter and the urine bag attached to the thigh, I find it difficult to sleep with it in place and wanted to avoid the discomfort when removed. The TURP procedure is relatively fast and is performed as same day surgery with usually very good results. The problem with the TURP for BPH is that it may need to be repeated if the prostate continues to enlarge with age (as it tends to do). Finally, while TURP may eliminate some cancer cells if there is malignancy in the prostate, it is really not one of the basic treatments for prostate cancer. Having a TURP for a BPH condition may also interfere with other forms of treatment for prostate cancer, which may be needed at a later time. As new procedures become available, the restrictions on the use of a TURP due to cancer treatments may not be as critical as once thought. More significant is that I was informed that the TURP often has to be repeated after a few years due to the prostate gland continuing to grow.

Infections

As I soon was to discover, there are other problems related to the prostate that can coexist with prostate cancer. Most of these are infections lumped under a general label, "prostatitis." The symptoms can be virtually the same as BPH and advanced prostate cancer and only careful examination can decide what you have.

Prostatitis usually is divided into two categories depending upon whether a bacterial infection or nonbacterial infection has caused the condition. In either event, prostatitis can become chronic. The only way the urologist can differentiate the two conditions is to take a urine sample and test for signs of bacteria or other causes. Most of the time both conditions are treated with antibiotics. Unfortunately, chronic bacterial prostatitis is just as its name indicates: a recurrent disorder with repetitive incidents. Nonetheless, even if a chronic problem is suspected, additional tests may be required if the condition continues after treatment in order to determine whether there is something else involved. There may be causes other than a bacterial or nonbacterial infection of the prostate and these include everything from nonbacterial irritation to sexually transmitted diseases.

The danger of prostatitis is not so much in its existence, but in the tendency for urologists and physicians to over-diagnose it. I personally can attest to this potential. When my PSA came back at 11.5 in December 1997 and at 0.72 in April 1998, the physician informed me that I probably had some form of prostatitis in December. This diagnosis also fitted nicely into the fact that the December biopsy had been negative and left me feeling warm and fuzzy!

If you are beginning to understand that this small walnut shaped gland can be the source of any number of problems you are correct. Unlike women who are made keenly aware of each aspect of their reproductive system, men generally continue to have no idea of the trouble this gland can cause them: prostate cancer; BPH; prostatitis of all types and variation; and interference with normal urinary function. At the risk of being repetitive, periodic examinations can go a long way to nip the problem in the bud. As a patient, the need to question and insist on getting to the bottom of the problem is critical. Do not take "no" for an answer. It is so easy to accept the lesser of evils as the cause of a problem without really knowing whether that it what you have. If the physician is reluctant to seek additional explanations for a recurrent problem, you absolutely need to secure a second opinion. This requires you to overcome the usual male hesitation to ask questions concerning urinary or sexual issues. Prostatitis may be caused by many bacteriological causes that only very specialized cultures of the urine specimen may indicate, such as parasites or even candida. Men need to get over their macho image and be forthright with their physician. Realistically, if you do not feel "right" now is not the time to "tough it out!"

PIN

Just when I believed I had learned just about everything any man needed to know concerning what could go wrong with my prostate I discovered there was another potential disorder. While this potential problem was one of academic interest, more than a present concern, it did raise some critical questions for all men namely, about what time in life does prostate cancer start? Of great importance is the fact that prostate cancer is being found in earlier stages due to better and earlier diagnosis. Emphasis is being placed more and more on attempting to locate biological "markers" indicating changes in the prostate which may take place before hard evidence of a malignancy is observable. There has developed a strong belief amongst many physicians that a condition called Prostatic Intraepithelial Neoplasia ("PIN") may well be a precursor to prostate cancer. Additionally, this condition does not appear to be called the same thing by all urologists, a factor which has added to the confusion as to what is the significance of PIN and its connection to future prostate cancer, if any.

What I was able to discern is that while there is no definitive proof that the presence of PIN is the same as the presence of prostate cancer, there is very persuasive evidence of some form of relationship between the two. Studies indicate that there appears to be a parallel between the ages when prostate cancer occurs and the presence of PIN. This can be important to the patient because prostate cancer seems to develop between twenty to thirty years after the onset of PIN. As is taking place in all areas of earlier cancer diagnosis, if you can pick up the "markers" of the disease early, then theoretically you should be able to nip the disease in the bud. A problem relates to this lag time between PIN and prostate cancer. If we assume the usual testing for prostate cancer starts around 50 years of age, does this mean we should be testing for prostate cancer at ages 20 or 30? Assuming this even makes sense, then what and how do we accomplish the test? PIN is determined the same way the physician discovers prostate cancer: the DRE and the biopsy! What if the patient does not have a high PSA? Does this mean he does not have PIN? Furthermore, PIN is divided into grades. There is a low grade and a high grade PIN. What is the significance at age 20 or 30 to having a low grade PIN versus a high grade PIN? In this regard, there are some similarities between the types of PIN to the Gleason Score used in grading the aggressiveness of prostate cancer. What is becoming more evident is that younger men are being diagnosed with the disease. It is no longer unusual to find men in their late thirties and early forties with Prostate Cancer. Whether this is the result of better diagnostic techniques or a more informed population is not clear. More studies will be needed over a protracted period to ascertain the answers.

If you are not totally confused yet, let me add to scratching of your head. For the sake of discussion, let's assume that a young man has a high PSA, a negative biopsy and a high grade PIN. Now what? If a careful reexamination of the biopsy tissue still shows no evidence of prostate cancer, then a program of careful watching and re-testing probably makes sense. New diagnostic techniques such as the PET Scan may be an important weapon in the monitoring of this individual since its' greater ability to find malignancies at earlier stages then most other tests.

The basic problem with PIN is that at present, there is no known treatment for this disorder. Assuming however that there is a connection between PIN and prostate cancer, it may well be that some form of hormonal treatment may be effective. Like so many aspects of diagnosing prostate cancer, PIN may provide a long-term indication of things to come. Obviously more investigation is required to be absolutely certain of the connection between PIN and prostate cancer, but this does not mean that PIN should be ignored.

As I learned about PIN, I could not help but wonder whether a test for PIN when my PSA was 11.5 and the biopsy was negative could have detected the presence of my prostate cancer in December 1997 instead of November 1998. The problem is that the only way of ascertaining the presence of PIN is biopsy. Even if PIN was detected, the lack of a clear relationship between it and prostate cancer would have undoubtedly resulted in no different action being taken. As subsequent events illustrated, my PSA was rising rapidly between these two dates. What significance these eleven months will ultimately have in the long-term prognosis of my disease has yet to be determined. Once again, the age-old adage that knowledge is power becomes more obvious.

Chapter 11

Staging the Disease

The doctor has received back the results of all of your diagnostic tests. The week or so of waiting has been one of uncertainty. Finally you have been told you have prostate cancer. The initial shock of the diagnosis takes time to absorb. You are just at the beginning of the fight. There is the need to find out as much as possible about the nature of your cancer and how advanced it may be. Prostate cancer, in spite of the fact it is slow growing, is a disease discovered in various stages of progression. The stage of the disease may well dictate the type and extent of treatment options that are best suited to deal with it.

My search became more intense and my feeling of some despair needed to be overcome. Just how advanced was my condition? Was I going to die in short order? I needed to understand the method of determining what the "stage" of my disease was. To some extent I didn't want to learn where I stood. There was no turning back at this juncture. I had prostate cancer and I needed to find out as much as I could as fast as I could. There was no sense in lying to myself. As an academic, my approach had to be to distance myself from myself and turn my research into a type of case study. It wasn't going to be easy.

Two systems exist that address the stages of prostate cancer. One system utilizes A, B, C, D and the other T1, T2, T3, T4, N, and M. In both systems, there are divisions in each category breaking down the various stages more exactly. Whether your physician uses one or the other makes little difference. Both systems follow similar gland sizes and the involvement of the cancer with surrounding tissue. After a diagnosis of the existence of prostate cancer, additional noninvasive tests such as MRI's, Cat Scans, and/or Bone Scans may be ordered to determine whether there has been a spread of the cancer beyond that of the prostate itself. Whether or not any of these additional diagnostic tests are ordered will often depend on the staging of the disease and the aggressiveness of the cancer.

I soon discovered that understanding the stage of the cancer, while not the complete picture, goes a long way to define the prognosis of the disease. The earliest stage where cancer is present in the prostate is stage "T1" or stage "A." The "T1" stage is further broken down into stage "T1a, T1b, and T1c." In all of the T1 stages, the presumption is that the cancer is located solely within the prostate gland and has not spread beyond it. It is important to recognize that this is a presumption, probably correct most of the time. Since microscopic extensions of the cancer outside of the gland edges do not cause symptoms and are not visible to MRI, CAT Scans, and/or Bone Scans, an absolute guarantee of encapsulation or organ confined, is not possible. Stage T1a or A1 is usually assigned to situations where the tumor is still too small to discover with the usual diagnostic techniques described earlier and, when found, the cancer is present in less then 5% of the biopsy sample taken from the gland.

Stage T1b or A2 defines a cancer where the biopsy sample contains more then 5% malignant tissue. You can have this stage of the disease even if other diagnostic tests have failed to indicate the location of the cancer. In this regard it is important to remember that the line of demarcation between Stages T1a-T1c can be relatively small.

Stage T1c or BO describes the discovery of cancer based upon a PSA with an elevated level and results in the taking of a biopsy. I have failed to fully understand the real significant differences between T1a and T1c other then the elevated PSA. In my diagnosis, the ultimate biopsy core sample in November 1998 came back indicating that less than 5% of the prostate tissue was malignant. Only two of eight samples were positive for the disease. Did this make my cancer a Stage T1a or a T1c? Did the difference have any long term bearing on my ultimate prognosis? Does it really matter what the Stage you are in as long as the tumor is still organ confined? The answer may be yes it does matter if you are to rely on a statistical chart developed by Dr. Partin discussed latter on in this book and set forth in the Illustrations portion of the Index.

My journey towards appropriate treatment and those of all men having been diagnosed with prostate cancer only begins once you have ascertained the stage of the disease. Staging the tumor is only part of the picture. The aggressiveness of the cancer was still not known. This information is needed before any form of treatment could be undertaken intelligently.

Although most men in today's medical environment will be found within the early stages of the disease, you need to be aware of the other stages as well. Once the tumor proceeds into stage T2, there usually is a clear ability on the part of the physician to feel something within the prostate gland during a digital rectal examination. The gland may feel lumpy or uneven. This may be evidence of a palpable tumor or of calcification caused by some other problem such as a chronic prostititus.

Stage T2a or B1N is usually located within one side (lobe) of the prostate. Within that side, the tumor is still small enough to be confined to less than one half of the side of the gland and generally less then 1.5 cm in size. It is very important to recognize that these early staging diagnoses are subject to revision. This is especially true in the case of removal of the gland. At that point of time, further biopsy of the gland may indicate that the initial evaluation was not correct. The pathologist may find that the cancer was more or less involved in the prostate than initially staged.

Stage T2b or B1 describes a tumor that is also palpable (able to be felt) but has spread to involve more than one half of one side of the prostate. The extension of the tumor into a larger area of the gland may not cause any symptoms, even at this point in time. That is a further reason to recognize that only through the periodic examination process can the cancer be discovered.

Stage T2c or B2 reflects the extension of the tumor into both sides of the prostate and is palpable during a digital rectal examination.

Both T1 and T2 are stages that an individual would like to be in when the cancer is discovered. Both, (subject to the presumption of that the cancer is still within the prostate), indicate no apparent spread of the disease and, in theory, offer the best hope for its long-term cure or control.

Stages T3 and T4 or C represent a more advanced stage, where the disease has spread outside of the prostate gland and become involved with other areas of the pelvic region. The disease is far more advanced. This does not mean that the disease is not treatable. What is involved at this stage, however, is a tumor that has probably been around for a longer period of time and may require more aggressive treatments.

T3 is a tumor that is easily felt through a digital rectal examination and has extended through the wall of the prostate gland. Surrounding tissue, including possibly the seminal vesicles, are also involved. Refining the staging somewhat, T3a or C1 indicates that the cancer on one side of the prostate gland has spread beyond the gland itself. Your physician may describe this as a "unilateral extracapsular extension." Regardless of the label, the cancer has breached the wall of the gland and is involved elsewhere.

Stage T3b or C2 is similar to stage T2c in that the tumor is located on both sides of the prostate gland and has spread beyond both sides of the walls of the gland. In stage T3c or C3, the cancer has involved either of the seminal vesicles or possibly both.

Stage T4a has no direct correlation to the other staging system of A, B, C, and D. Some diagnosticians will who utilize the A, B, C, and D staging will sometimes extend the C category slightly to encompass T4a. The real concern in a stage T4a environment is that the disease may have already spread to areas immediately surrounding the prostate, such as the rectum, the external bladder sphincter, bladder neck and pelvic lymph nodes. At this point there may be the inability to urinate properly, dependent upon the extent of the disease spread.

Stage T4b may now be in the pelvic wall as well as in certain structures known as the "levator muscles." You need to understand that situations as bad as some of these latter staging may appear, treatment options are still available to address the disease. The real significance of stage T3 and T4 disease is that additional treatment options may come into play that may or may not be needed to be utilized in earlier stages.

Once the disease is advanced to stage T3 and T4 there is greater involvement and possibly distant beyond the pelvic region of the body such as, into the lymph system, bones, and other bodily organs. This does not mean that the pelvic lymph nodes can't be involved at any stage of the disease. When it spreads beyond the pelvic region, prostate cancer appears quite often in the spine, hips, thighbones, and ribs. At this juncture the patient has very obvious symptoms including, but certainly not limited to: bone pain, fatigue, and weight loss.

At the risk of appearing repetitive, with periodic examinations, no man should be diagnosed for the first time with prostate cancer that is into these latter stages, or even T3 or T4. The reason should be self-evident. The more advanced the stage of the disease, the more difficult it is to treat, and the less optimistic the prognosis. At present there are few effective treatments for later stage metastasized prostate cancer. This does not mean that all is lost, since new treatments are evolving on almost a weekly basis. However, the earlier the detection of prostate cancer, the better is the over-all chances for effective treatment. This continues to lead to a belief on the part of some urologists that men need to be examined at earlier ages espe-cially as younger men are being diagnosed with the disease.

Staging the disease is not an exact science. The earliest and the late stages of the disease may provide the largest consensus for the stage, but the majority of the men will fall into the so-called early stages that may or may not be viewed the same way by different physicians. When first diagnosed I was informed that I had a "very early stage" since the examining physi-cian could not visualize any tumor on a MRI, CAT Scan or internal ultra-sound. His conclusion was that I was a "Stage T1b."

Upon seeking out a second opinion at an equally prestigious medical cen-ter, the examining physician told me that I could have a "Stage T2," since nothing was visualized. Since the prostate cancer was only was discovered through the biopsy, this second physician further confused the issue by stating that "the entire gland might have small clusters of malignant cells that had already extended beyond the capsule of the gland." I will never know which physician was correct or for that matter whether their differ-ences in opinion would have altered the methods of treatment I ultimately underwent. What I hoped to ascertain from this staging process was that my cancer was "organ confined" and my chances for "cure" were good. After being told I had an early stage, I was yet to find comfort since more diagnostic statistics were to be thrown my way. The problem is that the more statistics are explained to the patient, the less likely you are to understand the nuances of the differences in the staging, except if you are at the extreme opposite ends of the statistical curve.

Chapter 12

Gleason Scores

I must be candid. Even though it has been explained to me and I have independently researched the matter, I am still not certain how uniformly diagnosed the Gleason scores are. In the Index to this book you can find a generalized representation of the differences in cellular structure utilized to vary the Gleason Scores. Looking at the "overlapping" areas of different cellular configuration I can see how several pathologists can come to different scores. Having said that, the Gleason scores are widely utilized in order to attempt to measure the "aggressiveness" of the prostate cancer. Not all prostate cancers are alike. Some are more virulent than others are. "Gleason Scores" tries to place them in a category that may affect both the treatment undertaken and the prognosis of the disease, especially when coupled with the PSA level.

The Gleason Grading System is based upon a scale of 1 to 5. Once the biopsy has been taken a pathologist examines the biopsy sample and proceeds to evaluate the progression of the cancer by the changes in the prostate cells from the normal to the abnormal. A representation of this progression can be seen in Illustration Number 8 in the Appendix. In theory, the lower the Gleason score, the less aggressive the prostate cancer. This lower score should translate into an overall better prognosis. The prostate cancer cells are graded by comparison to the normal prostate cells. The closer the cancer cells resemble the normal tissue, the lower the Gleason score. For example, a Gleason score of "1" would indicate that the cancer cells resemble the normal prostate tissue very closely. The cancer cells are close together with well-defined shapes and most closely resemble normal prostate tissue.

As you progress to Gleason "2," the cancer cells are also close together, but there may be irregular spacing between the cells with some of the cells invading the surrounding muscle. In reality, Gleason 1 and 2 scores are very rare.

Gleason "3" (sometimes divided in 3a, 3b, 3c) illustrates cancer cells that are less defined and may even become cylindrical in form and shape. The Gleason "3" score is by far the most common finding of all.

In Gleason "4" (sometimes divided into 4a and 4b), the cancer has changed shape to form large masses or chain-like links.

Gleason "5" (sometimes divided into 5a and 5b), shows cells that have become solidified or clumped together. An important factor you need to keep in mind is that each increase in the Gleason score is more than merely one level higher. The higher the score, the greater is the risk of a poor prognosis.

As I have discovered in discussions with various pathologists, it is very common for the prostate to contain cancerous cells that are very different from each other and fall into different Gleason grades. Because of these variations, the final basis of the scoring is a combination of biopsy specimens. As specimens are examined under the microscope, the pathologist adds together the two most commonly found types of cancer cells and arrives at a total score. If there are two samples where one scores as a "2" and the other a "4," the total Gleason score would be a "6." The lower the total score, the slower the cancer is presumed to be growing. If you are lucky enough to have a grade 2 to 4, you are generally believed to have a tumor with slow progression. Scores of 5 to 6 are viewed as intermediate grades, while 7 to 10 are deemed aggressive and the prognosis is more serious. Some literature on Gleason Scores will state that the "primary and secondary scores are added together." In any event, the total score is the one that gives the sum utilized to aid in defining the prognosis of the disease. Understandably, if the Gleason Score comes back as a "7" or higher, you may develop as sense of despair. You haven't even decided on the best treatment for you and you cannot give into panic if the Gleason score is high. Conversely you cannot feel overly relieved if the score is low. Statistics are just that! In the long-term prognosis of any cancer, there are no definitive answers. I have a friend who is a clergyman, diagnosed with a Gleason Score of "8" whose father had died some years back from prostate cancer. Without disclosing the treatment he selected, he is doing fine with a post treatment PSA level of under 0.1! This individual is now six years past his treatment and his PSA has still not varied from the 0.1 level.

It is often recommended that you might want a second opinion on the Gleason Score findings. As many men soon discover if they decide to take the pathology report and samples to another pathologist the results can be more alarming. In my case, the Gleason score read by the pathologist at a major New York City Medical Center was "3 + 3 = 6." Although there was not much verbiage on the report, there was a sufficient amount to indicate that in the two samples from the biopsy that were positive, the pathologist found a consistency in both samples, which formed the basis of his findings. At the recommendation of a radiologist, (who warned me that another pathologist might read the results higher and rarely lower), I went to another equally large New York City medical center. The second pathologist came back with a total Gleason Score of "7." There was no differentiation between the two samples; only a final grade. The verbiage was unsettling. The second pathology report stated bluntly that I had a "most aggressive cancer of the virulent type." How could two respected institutions, which have performed prostate cancer evaluations thousands of times for very large urology departments, be so far apart in their respective analysis? Were there ulterior motivations behind these differences? I suspect that the latter question was borne more from my confusion than any evil intent on anyone's part. Once again however, the variations in diagnosis of scoring underlines that problems confronting the individual attempting to get a handle on what is happening to their body. I also suspect that most people will prefer to accept the lower staging and the lower Gleason Score in an attempt to lessen their fears and apprehensions concerning their disease! You need to be honest with yourself at all times while going through the process of diagnosis and treatment. Do not wish for what does not exist! Face up to the problem and do not give in to panic or despair. You have a long path to tread ahead of you and you need to keep a clear head.

Chapter 13

Partin Tables

Having gathered all of the diagnostic information the issue I had to face up to was putting all of the PSA, Staging and Gleason Scores together, now what? Was I now at that point where I could make intelligent choices for my treatment? Did I know enough? Was I involved with information overload? All of these questions will confront any man who has been diagnosed with prostate cancer.

The answer to these questions led to a further statistical maze known as the Partin Coefficient Tables. The Tables are set forth in the Illustrations Index of the Appendix to this book. I had gradually come to grips with my diagnosis and had even developed a degree of comfort concerning the stage of my disease and my lack of symptoms. I was further heartened by the sense that the tumor was neither visible by MRI, CAT SCAN nor physically palpable. Whether that view of my diagnosis was justified or not, I had come to peace with my pathology! I had a high PSA, 13.5, a Gleason 6, and probably a stage T1c. Then I got hit with the Partin Table prognosis. These Tables are probability-based and are used to predict the chances of the prostate cancer being organ-confined. The prognosis does change when the prostate cancer has escaped the organ itself and spread beyond into the surrounding tissue or lymph system. The Partin Table told me that I had a 38% chance of the cancer having spread beyond the capsule of the gland. If I were to believe the second pathologist's report of Gleason 7, my chances that the cancer had spread beyond the capsule was 45%. So much for the comfort level! At this juncture for the first time since my diagnosis, I came close to becoming depressed.

Before you panic, once you learn what the odds are for the spread of the disease, it is important to remember how subjective statistical diagnosis can be. Every diagnostic test is subject to variability. As any one may recall from high school or college statistics, probability theories are dependent upon the population sample and the uniformity of the collection of the data that goes into the calculation. View all of these statistical factors as merely pieces of information to be put into a proper perspective. It is so easy to become caught in the emotional swing of hope and despair as each piece of information is acquired. Statistics deal with numbers. You are an individual.

While the Gleason Score does have a proximate relationship to the treatment many urologists prefer, the Partin Tables project potential prognosis. It is for this reason that having confidence in the Gleason scoring is critical. Did I feel uneasy about the vast difference in the readings of my biopsy? Did the higher reading affect my decision concerning the type of treatment I settled upon? In all probability, the higher score did not have an impact on the treatment decision, but only because I had been forewarned that different pathologists might apply different subjective interpretations to the biopsy samples. If you take a close look at the Illustrations in the Index indicating the various stages utilized for arriving at the Gleason Score, it becomes apparent that in borderline Gleason Score cases, it may become difficult to identify the true Partin score. Keep in mind, If you change the Gleason score, then the Partin Table results change!

In the long run, after much research and questioning, I am not certain what the significance is of the Partin Table for a single case. Disease has a way of doing what it wants to do without much regard for gross statistics. On an individual basis, an individual may or may not confirm the statistics.

The Partin Table, at least on the surface, does not take into account other variables such as familial history of prostate cancer, the age of the individual, or the environment. In the latter variable, it is interesting to note that the U.S. Department of Veteran Affairs has recently related military service in Vietnam with prostate cancer to the extent that it is now recognized as a service connected disorder. What factors could possibly give rise to this determination except for the environmental conditions within which the military served? The environmental condition, which comes to mind, is the wide use of Agent Orange, the subject of much litigation and medical investigation.

As more prostate cancer statistics are gathered, other statistical tables will undoubtedly come into existence, which may or may not substantiate the Partin Tables. View the Partin Tables in the Index of this book intelligently and without a sense of panic or doom. When I went to another medical institution to evaluate my biopsy report, I was both amused and concerned when the urologist took out of his pocket a small card—the Partin Tables—and proceeded to inform me of the seriousness of my disease. When questioned as to whether any procedure over any other would alter the Partin statistical outcome, he had no answer.

Diagnosis of your prostate condition depends on the totality of many tests and the ability of your physician together with yourself to piece the entire puzzle together. The tremendous advantage you possess is that in most cases, prostate cancer gives you sufficient time to make intelligent decisions and to absorb as much information as possible. Give yourself a break. Don't bury yourself or listen to those who haven't done their homework. Review the diagnostic tests with professionals who can explain what they mean and how you can you best evaluate the next step—your treatment. Your treatment is related to the diagnostic tests you have undertaken and the results from them. It is at this juncture that the MRI's, CAT SCANS, Bone Scans, PSA, PSA II, Gleason Scores, all come together as you face the next step in the process of your care.

In July 2004, a series of articles appeared in the New England Journal of Medicine that addressed another measuring device for ascertaining the potential of reoccurrence of the disease after the surgical removal of the prostate gland. The authors looked at the "rate of increase" in the PSA levels prior to treatment. These physicians appear to believe that the rate of PSA increases prior to diagnosis can by itself indicate the grade of the tumor and the stage of the disease. Their study would seem to show that an increase in the PSA of 2.0 or more per year prior to diagnosis was significant regardless of the Gleason Score or the Partin Table Statistics.

In the same issue of the New England Journal of Medicine, Dr. Partin [of Partin Table fame] appeared to suggest that there may in fact be some validity to the rate of increase prior to diagnosis. The real question of course still has to be whether this finding holds true for all men faced with a rapid increase of PSA levels, or is it merely another statistical factor to be weighed in determining the ultimate treatment for the management of the disease. What becomes more confusing for the man diagnosed with prostate cancer has to be how to deal with all of the statistical factors with which he finds himself confronted?

I must admit upon reading the recent studies and in light of my own history of rapid increases in my PSA prior to diagnosis, the initial reaction was that I was going to die from prostate cancer and that perhaps all of the treatment I had undergone was a waste of time, energy, money and emotion. Yet, I have gone over seven years since my last treatment and my PSA continues to fall. The last test in August 2006 was 0.15. This, together with a considerably diminished prostate gland, has provided me with a degree of reassurance. Does this mean that I am cured and I no longer have to concern myself with follow-ups? Clearly the answer is "no!" Unlike many other cancers, prostate cancer tends to have a timetable all its own, with years of potential uncertainty for the man diagnosed with the disease. What I have learned is to master the situation rather then to have the situation master me.

PART II

TREATMENT

Chapter 14

General Treatment Options

There are so many various treatments for prostate cancer. Some are "main stream" and some are clearly innovative and experimental. Although I was intrigued by the new innovative treatments many are so far from being proven that I tended to discount them as being far too uncertain. As a result the treatments described here are only those that have generally been utilized in the main stream of medical practice. This does not mean that others out in the marketplace or on the drawing boards well may hold significant promise for the future. Since the writing of the original book, new treatments have been developed and/or refined. New experimental drugs have been tested, some seeking to prevent the disease and others to address reoccurrence. Drugs such as "finasteride" may hold a promise of preventing prostate cancer. In the recent results of a trial of the drug which has been conducted for the past seven years, it appeared that the finasteride reduced prostate cancer cases in the test group by 25 percent. There are side effects to the use of the drug that have raised some concerns. The best candidates for the drug appear to be men who are African-American and those with family histories of prostate cancer.

A new twelve year international study entitled "SELECT" is looking into the use of Vitamin E and selenium as a possible prevention of prostate cancer.

The options for treatment of prostate cancer have increased greatly over recent years. The reasons have been the result of several factors. Foremost has been a better understanding of the range of disease progression and recognition that not every treatment appears to make sense for each stage of the disease. In some instances, more consideration must be given to the age of the man afflicted and his life expectancy. Fundamentally troublesome with utilizing age, as a consideration is that actuary tables no longer have the validity they once possessed. Men are living longer and are healthy well into old age. Many formerly fatal disorders are being controlled through new treatments and medications. While it may be comforting to state that the average man of 75 will probably outlive his prostate cancer, more and more 75 years olds in otherwise good health are living well into their 80's. Longer life requires a rethinking of utilizing age as a sole criterion for treatment modalities. This is especially apparent if the man suffering from prostate cancer is in otherwise good health.

What is good health? Even the definition of good health is a relative term, since few individuals reach their 70's without some disorder. Life expectancies have lengthened considerably in the Western World over the last one hundred years, and this trend seems to be continuing. The 75-year-old today may still be alive and vital ten to fifteen years from now! The 60-year-old may have 25 more years of productive living! Productive living gives rise to the issue of "quality of life." So long as a person has an acceptable quality of life as that individual defines the term, age may be the least of the criteria to be considered. This being the case, age is merely one factor in the type of treatment to be considered by the man diagnosed with prostate cancer. More critical to the determination of the treatment may be the degree to which the treatment may alter the perception of the man and his relationship to those around him. As I indicated earlier in this book, continual vigilance is critical to maintaining good health. Men even in their 70's need to be tested annually to make certain the treating physician can establish "base line" PSA levels in order to monitor increases.

After all is said and done there are approximately six basic approaches to the treatment of prostate cancer along with certain variations within some of them. Each one carries its own unique set of advantages and disadvantages. Some of the treatments have been around longer than others. As new studies seem to indicate, the so-called tried and true approach may not necessarily be as much of a "sure thing" as was once believed. There are as many studies and reports on each approach to treatment as there are members of the Congress of the United States! If you decide to review a selected number of them you would soon ascertain that they tend to have a built in bias. Physicians are partial to what makes them comfortable. The medical researchers often base their conclusions as to the effectiveness of one treatment over another on analytically diversified methods. Trying to compare different conclusions becomes one of the most frustrating problems confronting men attempting to determine what is the correct path for them to take. Comparisons often are difficult, if not impossible.

New techniques and theories appear to be constantly evolving. Variations in the basic treatments all sound impressive. A warning to any new treatment must be sounded, since the disease tends to have such a long progression. A new treatment may take at least ten to fifteen years to fully evaluate. Further many of the studies that compare various forms of treatment, I am sorry to state, come from the predilection of a medical center or physician for particular forms of treatment. It is so important to understand that no treating physician can ever state with surety that a given procedure "will be a guaranteed cure for the problem." If any physician makes this statement to you, seek another opinion immediately. I found myself in this exact predicament when I was told "at your age and at your stage of the disease, we can perform surgery and you'll be cured and over with it!" There were no other options that this physician would consider. I pressed him as to the side effects of surgery and received a long discourse on how limited they were. Further if side effects did occur, "I have perfected a subsequent procedure to correct them." I needed another physician who would be willing to explain to me the options and the associated risks along with the probabilities of long-term success—in realistic terms.

Chapter 15

Surgery

There is no getting around the fact that surgery has been the mainstay of prostate cancer treatment for several years. The philosophy in the treatment of cancer has been traditionally to remove the disease from the body by cutting out the cancer along with surrounding tissue, just in case there might be any microscopic spread that could not be seen by the surgeon. The pathologist to ascertain whether there was indeed any spread of the disease would then examine the removed tissue. Further, the view of many a patient was that the only chance for a cure was through the actual surgical removal of cancer. Surgery is therefore the first option considered by most men when told they have prostate cancer. An acquaintance of mine stated it bluntly, "it was cancer and I wanted it out of my body!" While urologists are setting out the alternatives to men, many have a clear preference to perform the surgery especially when the diagnostic tests come back indicating early stage disease.

Obviously, no patient likes surgery. The thought of one's body being cut open and invaded has always carried with it fear and uncertainty. Other than a hammertoe operation on my small toe and my tonsils being removed, both when I was a youngster, and some teeth extracted, I had not had a serious surgery. However, for the vast majority of urologists and patients alike, surgery is still held out as the preferred treatment for prostate cancer. Whether surgery provides a better rate of survival is one of the most debated issues in the treatment of prostate cancer. One of the most troublesome factors to be considered in the leap to undergo surgery is the belief that by removing the cancerous prostate, the individual is cured of the disease. This may be true, but the assumption one must make is that there is no microscopic spread of the disease outside of the capsule of the gland. Statistics can be troublesome since they seem to indicate that this may not be true over the long haul.

Radical Surgery

If you decide to undergo radical surgery you need to know how the procedure is performed and all of the associated ramifications. Surgery for removal of the cancerous prostate is not a simple procedure. I have found in my discussions with a number of urologists that many find it easy to downplay the fact that this is a major abdominal procedure if performed in the retropubic manner. It is also a bloody operation, and most men are advised to donate at least two pints of their own blood in advance of the surgery. Although much headway has been made in the inspection of blood for serious diseases, you do have the time to prepare for the surgery. This adds an additional margin of safety for the patient.

There are two basic techniques for radical surgical removal of the prostate gland. The most commonly utilized is the retropubic, which performs surgery through an incision in the lower abdomen. An Illustration in the Index indicates where the incision is usually made.

The second and less frequently utilized method for removal of the prostate gland is the perineal approach. In this procedure, the gland is removed by an incision made between the testicles and the anus. An Illustration in the Index indicates where the incision is usually made.

A third surgical procedure may be utilized to examine the lymph nodes when the perineal surgical procedure has been utilized. This requires what is known as a laparoscopic lymphadenectomy and requires incisions to be made in the area of the belly button. The perineal surgery due to the location of the incision does not allow for the pelvic lymph nodes to be examined during the procedure.

Retropubic surgery involves making an incision in the front of the lower abdomen that provides the surgeon with the best overall view of the area. The entire gland is removed along with associated tissue and the seminal vesicles. The urethra normally has to be temporarily severed from the bladder during the procedure and then reattached after the gland has been removed. The pelvic lymph nodes are accessible in this procedure. Most surgeons will remove the pelvic lymph nodes in order to biopsy them to ascertain if there is any spread of the cancer. Historically, in the process of the removal of the prostate gland and surrounding functions, the nerves that control the erectile function of the penis are also intentionally removed or accidentally damaged in the process of the actual surgery. More often than not, this leads to impotence. Although subsequent use of drugs such as Viagra may return erectile function, there is no guaranty. The technique for this surgery has been improved in recent years through a procedure pioneered by Dr. John Walsh of Johns Hopkins Medical Center. The surgery attempts to spare the nerves that control the erectile function of the penis. It would be foolish to believe that the loss of potency is not a problem. The loss of potency has a tremendously negative psychological effect on most men. In a society that has created the "macho" image, the inability to perform sexually can be as serious a problem as the cancer itself. Viagra may not be for everyone and in fact may be dangerous for some men with coronary problems. Additionally, Viagra is expensive and many men cannot afford such an expensive drug. Therefore, to the extent that these nerves can be spared, a fuller quality of life may be able to be continued in many men.

The procedure for the surgical removal of the prostate utilizing the retropubic procedure requires between three to five days stay in the hospital. As is the case with all surgery, there is associated discomfort and pain. The surgery requires the use of a catheter inserted in the penis to drain the bladder while the patient is healing from where the urethra was sewn back to the bladder. Most urologists will leave the catheter in for up to 14 days. I have heard of men having the catheter in place for as long as 21 days. Although a friend of mine indicated that he went to work with the catheter in place and a urine collection bag attached to the front of his thigh, I suspect that he was either crazy or in the minority of men. The catheter is uncomfortable at best, and at worst downright irritating. I still recall what I thought was the macabre humor of my urologist when he discussed putting a catheter back into me and stated how easy a procedure it was—for him! It was the last time I indicated that I was having some painful urination. He wasn't being funny.

The actual recovery time at home will vary from person to person. Most urologists seem to feel that within about five weeks, you should be able to resume your life. However, stretching, bending, and lifting carries the risks of the second potential side effect to this surgery, hernia. Statistics are wonderful when you happen to be the individual with whom everything goes well. The fact remains that many men will suffer from urine leakage or urgency problems requiring frequent urination after the surgery. A percentage will never fully recover total bladder control and will be required to wear some form of control underwear for the rest of their lives. The radical procedure may also cause erectal dysfunction. Even with the nerve sparing operation, a small survey indicates that between 17% to 32% of men suffered some form of urinary leakage.

Impotence and incontinence are the twin risks to the quality of life after the surgery. What is most troubling is that both problems are difficult to assess accurately, partly due to the reluctance of patients to discuss them with their physician. In many situations involving older men these problems have developed prior to the onset of prostate cancer. Even younger men may have these problems caused by other health problems. Impotence and incontinence are serious side effects to the surgery and if you contemplate surgery as your treatment you must understand these risks. A survey of Medicare patients who underwent surgery in the period 1988-1990 indicated that urinary wetness required 30% of the men to use pads or even clamps and 63% of all patients had current problems with wetness. While other studies tend to indicate different results, discussions with many men who have undergone the radical procedure seems to be in line with the Medicare study. However, a friend of mine summed up his attitude (and I suspect the attitude of many men) by informing me that he didn't mind leaking or failing to achieve an erection so long as the "damn cancer was out of my system!" As an aside it is interesting to note that he recently discussed with me the many procedures he has been experimenting with in order to achieve an erection.

There is an older and still utilized surgical technique, which seeks to spare the patient some of the potential discomfort and risks of abdominal surgery: perineal prostatectomy. This surgery is performed by making an incision between the testicles and the anus. While the same cancerous prostate is removed through this approach, the lymph nodes cannot be reached readily. If there is a suspicion or a desire to examine the lymph nodes, then a separate procedure is necessary. It is also harder to spare the nerves. Recovery time and all other factors are the same between the two procedures including the insertion of a catheter and the length of time it must be in place. The risks of incontinence and impotence are about the same for both procedures.

Surgery is not for everyone, regardless of age. As a general rule, surgery is performed on men who are younger, (usually less than seventy years of age), in good general health, and appear to have early stage disease. It is very important to recognize that even when the prostate cancer appears to be contained within the gland that does not guarantee that there is no microscopic spread of the disease beyond the capsule. It is also important to recognize that many physicians believe it is not essential to perform a bone scan and/or MRI when the Gleason Score is 6 or below, the PSA is 10 or less, and the cancer is T1a, 1b or 1c. Don't listen! Insist on these tests even if you have to pay for them yourself. They may provide further evidence of disease or relative peace of mind indicating no spread of the disease. Always remember it is your body. If necessary, make a pest of yourself!

As unsettling as it may appear even with radical surgery, a relatively large number of patients develop further disease years later. This may be caused by a failure to discover microscopic extensions of the tumor or an understating of the stage of the disease when originally diagnosed. The statistics again vary from study to study, however, 25% to 28% of patients will require follow-up treatment at some point after the surgery has been performed.

For many men, the extent of the disease is not fully known unless a reoccurrence takes place. Some will discover that the cancer has already spread when the pathologist analyzes the tissue following surgery. Others will be told that there was no evidence of any spread of the disease in surrounding tissue and therefore they are cured! A little shock reality is needed here. The word "cure" may exist when the optimum conditions seem to prevail. However, you will not be completely certain that you are cured until probably fifteen years have past since the surgery. Dependent upon your age and general health, some other disaster or illness may overtake you before a recurrent prostate cancer appears.

It is the policy in many institutions where retropubic prostatectomy is performed not to proceed further with the operation until the lymph nodes have examined. If the pelvic lymph nodes indicate presence of the disease, the surgeon does not proceed further. In this situation the patient is referred to other forms of treatment such as radiation or hormone therapy. Be certain to ask your physician, if you choose surgery what procedure he recommends if the pelvic lymph nodes come back positive. Have him explain in detail why the prostate is not removed and what particular treatment will then be undertaken—and when?

Cryosurgery—Temperature-Monitored Cryoablation of the Prostate

There is still one other form of surgery that should be discussed in order to provide the fullest range of options to the patient: cryoablation or temperature-monitored target cryoablation of the prostate (TCAP). I must be candid in that I did not consider this option as a possible treatment. I was never informed of its existence by any of the physicians with whom I spoke, and found only passing references to this treatment in all of my investigations. Nevertheless, this procedure has been utilized for other tumors in the body for years and has been utilized in the treatment of prostate cancer for more than five years.

One of the advantages of TCAP is that it may be utilized even after other forms of prostate cancer treatments have been performed and may be repeated after it has been used. It appears that this surgical treatment is available for individuals who may not be in the best of general health, of older age, or who have been diagnosed with disease that has spread beyond the gland. To date, there does not appear to have been much use of this treatment with younger men with lower grade prostate cancers.

The patient can be sedated either through general anesthesia or by a spinal. Much like the seed implantation procedure, six to eight cyroprobes are inserted in the perineal region (between the testicles and anus) using a transrectal ultrasound as a guide. There are side effects and risks with the procedure. New temperature monitoring indicate the temperature necessary to be effective. At the same time a device is used to warm the urethra in order to avoid damage. There is danger of freezing the rectum and the urethra. New techniques for maintaining warmth in the urethra have lessened significantly the problems associated with earlier use of this procedure, but impotence and incontinence are potentially as significant as other surgeries. Men with large prostate glands due to natural physiology or conditions such as BPH may need to have the glands shrunk in order to make the region subjected to freezing a smaller target. This may require placing the patient on Lupron, Zoladex, Eulexin and/or Casodex over a short period of time in order to accomplish the reduction of the gland size.

As treatments for prostate cancer go, cryoablation has not developed the extent of statistical data that other treatments have amassed. At this juncture there is about ten years of data that appears very encouraging except for impotence. Eighty-five percent of the men undergoing this procedure become impotent. This does mean that this treatment is not valid. It may well be a better treatment than any other. Unfortunately, because prostate cancer tends to require long periods of time in order to ascertain the effectiveness of treatment, it may take years to evaluate fully whether this treatment will survive the test of time. What has been observed to date is that if the tumor is big and the cancer fairly involved, the use of this treatment does not appear to be as effective as might be desired. Animal experimentation has shown that utilizing freezing and microwave radiation in combination with each other may be more effective. In spite of the limitations and uncertainties concerning this treatment, cryoablation should be included in any discussion with your treating physician when determining what the best treatment for your situation may be. On a recent television show discussing cryoablation, the urologist indicated to the host he believed that in the long run this treatment would surpass all others presently being utilized for the treatment of prostate cancer. It is interesting that my own urologist as well as others who had been committed to other forms of treatment are utilizing cryoablation for primary and reoccurring prostate cancer with apparently excellent results.

In July 1999, the Federal Health Care Financing Administration determined that this procedure was a safe primary treatment option for localized prostate cancer. In effect this means that insurance companies will pay for the procedure.

The techniques for the performing this procedure have improved tremendously in recent years. One of the major problems in the past involved the regulation of the temperature of surrounding tissue near the prostate. Now a catheter is inserted into the urethra that is maintained at a predetermined warm temperature. Ultrasound pictures similar to those utilized for radioactive seed implantation, provide good imaging to locating the probe being inserted into the prostate gland. Although claims have been made that this procedure lessens the risk of incontinence, the risk of impotence is very high. What is also interesting to note is that cryosurgery can be repeated if necessary. The procedure has been utilized in cases of localized reoccurrence and where radiation therapy has not been effective.

Microwave

A newer approach to the treatment of prostate cancer has taken a page out of the primer on microwave oven operation. Just as your kitchen microwave cooks from the inside out through heating the cellular structure of food, so this concept has taken on an application for the treatment of prostate cancer. The effect is to cook the cancer, thus killing it and allowing the body mechanisms to remove the dead tissue internally.

Only recently recommended by its advisory committee to be approved by the Food and Drug Administration, a device called the Prostatron utilizes microwaves to destroy the prostate tissue. The device is inserted through a catheter to the prostate, which heats up and destroys the glandular tissue.

Assuming there will be final approval by the FDA, there are obvious issues that need to be addressed by the patient before undertaking this procedure. It is a new procedure with little history as to its success. Most important, does it destroy all of the cancer? Is it acceptable for all stages of the disease? What, if any, are the side effects of the treatment? Like cryosurgery, heat may adversely impact on the urethra, rectum and surrounding tissues. The treatment certainly would appear to have some application to BPH conditions by shrinking the gland to relieve symptoms. Perhaps that is where its ultimate benefit may be found.

Similar to microwave treatment is the use of lasers and ultrasound to destroy prostate tissue. The use of these procedures in the treatment of BPH has gained popularity since there appears to be less potential nerve damage then the traditional TURP. Although these latter treatments may not appear to be truly surgical, (as that term may be understood within the medical profession), all involve a degree of invasiveness carrying the potential for serious side effects. The advantage of these lesser known treatments is that they are more readily acceptable for individuals who may have other health problems which preclude the more invasive radical surgical procedures.

At the risk of appearing unduly repetitive, critical to any treatment decision, especially when considering radical surgery, is the effect it will have on the quality of life of the patient. A major consideration I had to make whether or not to have radical surgery was how would it interfere with my life style? As important to my decision was the fact that as an active man, who has always considered himself younger than his years, being incapacitated for a protracted period of time was not to my liking. This is not to say that I was willing to trade off the possibility of long term cure for present life style. My investigations were predicated on a balanced approach to what treatments were available and whether I deemed them satisfactory for my needs. Critical to any treatment decision has to be whether they carried with them the real possibility of a long-term survival? Personally I had no fear of cancer, viewing it as merely another disease that needed to be dealt with by myself in an intelligent manner. However, if you are an individual who has deep-seated fears of cancer and can only feel psychologically content if the diseased gland and surrounding tissue are removed, then surgery must be in the forefront of the treatment options you seek. This is one of the difficulties in assessing the appropriateness for each individual of treatment they ultimately will select. The treatment you will decide upon must be predicated upon both the stage of the disease, and also upon your own mental outlook.

Regardless of your personal views, surgery may in fact be the best approach to the treatment of the disease when viewed from the perspective of age, PSA, Gleason Scores, and longevity potential. Many physicians still prefer to suggest surgery for younger patients with early stage disease. To what extent studies such as those discussed early in this book (concerning rates of PSA increase prior to diagnosis) will have on treatment options is still not clear. If you truly believe some of the statistical tables and articles published by various medical institutions, surgery would apparently provide the best chance for long-term survival although more recent studies would seem to question these former premises. If surgery is the way you choose to proceed do not loose sight of the newer techniques which hold out the promise of fewer side effects and the hope for continued sexual function. If sexual function is not an issue, then the nerve sparing procedure may not be of critical importance. Remember that unlike other forms of cancer, you have some time to fully assess what is your best treatment. Do owe yourself the favor of not being panicked into any decision you may regret later on! Of equal importance, once you feel comfortable with the decision you have made concerning treatment,

DO NOT LOOK BACK! Do not second-guess the decision you have made—it can drive you crazy. Anecdotal stories from friends and neighbors about their preferred treatment or, those of relatives should not rattle you. Unless you know everything about the other persons' disease, no two people are alike. It comes down to—your choice, your body.

ROBOTIC SURGERY

The surgical removal of the prostate through the use of robotic surgery is starting to be utilized by some hospitals in the United States. Pioneered by the United States Government, remote surgery for battlefield injuries has entered the mainstream.

Small incisions are made in the pubic region and through the use of a laproscope the prostate is removed. The surgeon need not be in the operating theatre but can direct the entire procedure from an adjoining room utilizing a computer monitor and mechanical arms to perform the operation. Proponents of this new technique claim that the advantages over traditional surgery are less pain; less need for blood transfusions, and a shorter recovery period, often allowing the patient to go home the next day.

The major concern of most patients is whether this procedure will enable the surgeon to prevent incontinence and impotence. Some surgeons have expressed concern that the procedure may not be as successful in removing malignant prostates then more traditional surgeries. Nonetheless, Robotic surgery is being touted more and more as the preferred manner for removal of the prostate. Friends of mine have undergone this procedure recently and have been back to work in a very short period of time with little of the trauma associated with the more traditional prostate surgical approaches. It is still too early for either of my friends to know whether they are impotent or incontinent.

Chapter 16

Radiation

There is an alternative treatment for prostate cancer to either form of surgery. Radiation as utilized in the treatment of prostate cancer is a generic term that covers a multitude of treatments involving some form of radiation therapy. Various types of radiation may be put to use in combination with other forms of treatment, that do not involve radiation. The term "radiation" must also be clarified since there are various radioactive elements used as well as tremendous differences in the delivery system employed.

In the simplest terms, radiation therapy is divided into "external" and "internal." "External" radiation includes various types and formats. With the development of new equipment and the utilization of different forms of radioactive isotopes, the approach to "external" radiation treatment has changed dramatically over the past ten years. These changes have not only involved prostate cancer treatment, but also virtually all forms of cancers where radiation therapy is being prescribed. 3-D Conformal Beam Radiation, Conformal Proton Beam Radiotherapy and Intensity Modulated Radiotherapy (IMRT), all provide radiation therapy to the prostate and are examples of "external" radiation.

"Internal" radiation refers to implantation or small pellets called seeds or "brachytherapy." Even this therapy can be divided further into both the type of radioactive isotope used in the implanted seed and whether it is to permanently remain in the prostate or only temporarily. The radioactive isotope can be long or short acting.

External Beam Radiation

The use of external beam radiation therapy for the treatment of various types of cancers has been around for several years.

In the 1950's when my mother was diagnosed with breast cancer, the state-of-the-art after surgery was a course of treatment with colbalt-60. The affected area was painted with a grid and the radiation dose was directed at each area over a period of several sessions. Fortunately, both science and medicine have progressed since the 1950's and the availability of new approaches to radiation therapy has improved. Nonetheless, no form of radiation is selective. The radiation will affect healthy as well as malignant tissue. It is for this reason that much of the new technology has been directed at limiting the damage to the surrounding healthy tissue. Earlier use of nonconformal-beam radiation had the unfortunate result of destroying healthy tissue as well as the cancerous tissue. It also had problems in ascertaining the actual depth of the tumor being attacked as well as the extent of the area to be irradiated. A more serious issue was whether this radiation was also causing separate malignancies resulting from its damage to healthy tissue surrounding the cancer being attacked.

There was always the issue relating to the correct dosage to be used on the patient. This lack of understanding added to the potential for not destroying all of the cancer. If given after the surgical removal of the cancer, just where should the radiation be directed? In my mother's situation, seven years after a radical mastectomy and sixty colbalt-60 treatments, the cancer returned in the exact area where the breast had been removed and the cancer had been located. Clearly, neither the radical surgery nor the intense radiation had done its job. Radiation therapy had to wait until newer diagnostic techniques became available Fortunately, today newer techniques as well as the use of different isotopes have materially altered the use of radiation to treat all forms of cancer and especially, prostate cancer.

Conformal Proton Beam Radiation

External conformal proton beam radiation is one of the new radiation technologies that attempt to limit potential damage to surrounding tissue. The therapy seeks to "conform" the beam to the area in need of treatment, and, by limiting the area involved, there is a greater ability to deliver higher doses of radiation to the prostate. Conformal Proton Beam Radiation therapy is not available everywhere, although the concept has been around for several years. The major advantage to Conformal Proton Beam therapy is that it can be aimed in such a manner as to pass through healthy tissue with minimal damage if any, to reach and destroy the prostate cancer cells.

In order to be effective, however, there is an absolute need to create a three dimensional model of the prostate. Once again, new technologies have made this approach possible and workable. The use of a CT (computed tomography) Scan to create the three dimensions needed is aided by immobilizing the patient. This is essential in order to make certain that each day the radiation is given, the patient is in the exact position as when the CT Scan was originally taken. Most institutions using this technique construct a rigid form that is usually made out of PVC, a form of plastic similar to the pipe material found in most houses today, and placed around the body of the patient. Interestingly, when I underwent this treatment, no rigid form was utilized. Rather, the oncologist tattooed three areas along my pubic hairline with pin point blue dots. I attempted to diffuse the situation with humor and suggested the radiologist connect the dots and play tic-tac-toe. These markers became the focus points for the twenty-five external radiation treatments that I underwent. Regardless of the method utilized, once the three-dimensional scan having been made, the radiation oncologist is then able to outline the area to be radiated on the computer screen. Additional players are needed for this treatment namely a physicist and an individual called the dosimetrist. Together, a plan is devised as to the angle the proton beams are to enter and the dose of radiation to be delivered.

My introduction to the actual treatment room reminded me of a science fiction movie although a friend who had similar treatments stated he felt like the Frankenstein Monster. There is a flat table-like platform upon which the patient lies down. The immobilizing device is placed upon and/or around the patient or in my case, I was asked to lower my trousers enough so the tattoos could be visualized. The machine delivering the proton beam can be moved to deliver the appropriate dosage by rotating around the actual table. I was always fascinating by two facts, the use of what appeared to be two covers modeled after my prostate placed over the aperture where the radiation came out of the machine. Each was a mirror image of the other and was open in the middle. The machine usually started on my left side, then moved overhead, then to my right side then underneath. The treatment itself is not long, but continues on a daily basis for a number of days dependent upon whether this is to be the only treatment given or in conjunction with other therapies. The "set-up" takes longer then the treatment itself. Daily adjustments of the position of the patient may be required in order to make certain the proton beam is as precisely located as possible to deliver the dosage required. There is no sensation of the beam entering the body. The only awareness the patient has is the sound of the equipment as it moves or starts up and shuts down. Frankly, after awhile the procedure is downright boring! I developed a certain sense of the absurd about the entire procedure. Here I was a mature man with my trousers lowered with this machine rotating around me a though it was an alien from outer space sizing me up. I even named the machine—old creaky, due to the sound it made as it rotated. A good sense of humor goes a long way when you undergoing prostate cancer treatment!

There are generally few side effects to this therapy. Some individuals do develop urinary urgency, burning sensations when urinating, and some rectal irritation. The latter problem can be either constipation or diarrhea. Changes in the diet can assist in the relieving of the symptoms. Additional benefit may be had from warm baths. Most of the time, these side effects disappear within weeks after the end of the treatment. Fatigue can also accompany the use of radiation therapy regardless of the type or kind employed. Rest and pacing your daily life patterns can ease the effect of fatigue should that symptom appear.

In rare cases, some form of medication may be required to address some of the side effects and to alleviate their impact. Although I did not undergo "proton beam" radiation, after about the fourth week of my conformal radiation therapy I had some burning urination and some fatigue. None of these were debilitating. I do know of one individual with whom I discussed this therapy who also developed skin sensitivity in the area where the radiation was given. This too disappeared some six weeks after the therapy.

There is still one other side effect that needs to be understood—impotence. It is generic to all forms of long-term radiation therapy and seems to develop about two years or so after the therapy is given. I have questioned several radiologists about this problem and there are different theories concerning why this occurs in some men. I also suspect that some of the men who develop impotence after the fact may not have been potent prior to the treatment. Interesting as it may be, none of the urologists, radiologists, or general physicians with whom I discussed my diagnosis of prostate cancer ever asked the obvious question—"are you sexually active and do you presently have any erectile or similar difficulties?" I personally believe the reason why this question is not asked may be that many men, out of a sense of being macho or embarrassment, may not answer the queries honestly. If you are still sexually active, you owe it to yourself and your spouse or significant other to raise the issue of effect of any form of radiation therapy on your sex life. Evaluate the response you receive as part of your decisional process regarding appropriate therapy for your needs. After all the treatments have been received, your life will continue. It is helpful not to be confronted with after the fact conditions for which you are not prepared!

TomoTherapy

TomoTherapy is a new method for the delivery of radiation to the prostate. The TomoTherapy Hi-Art System is a new approach to radiation treatment of prostate cancer and other malignant tumors. This system delivers radiation in the form of a spiral pattern around the patient by having the machine rotate around a supine patient. The tumor can be targeted more accurately with less potential for damage to healthy tissues. Prior to each treatment the doctor is able to exactly redefine the location of the tumor. Most individuals are not aware of the fact that tumors can move and even change shape as a result of treatment. This new form of delivery of radiation can compensate for these movements allowing for refocusing of the beam. The ability of this new procedure to attack the tumor from 360 degrees should enable a more exact form of treatment. As is the case with any new technology, time will be the ultimate judge of its effectiveness.

Three Dimensional Conformal Radiation— (3D CRT)

In order to be effective, any radiation therapy has to deliver a sufficient dosage to kill the cancer in the intended area. In the case of prostate cancers, there are several sensitive body functions significantly close to the prostate gland. Unrestricted radiation therapy can do considerable damage to the rectum, bladder, urethra, and surrounding tissues. The higher the radiation dosage, the greater the risk of not only permanent injury, but also protracted side effects. While it is easy in the abstract to say, "I won't mind the side-effects so long as the cancer is destroyed," as I'll discuss in more detail, the side effects can be very unpleasant and can make your life miserable. With the parallel development of new computers and three-dimensional software coming together to enable new techniques to be undertaken in the field of radiation therapy, side effects may be able to be minimized.

If you ask your children or grandchildren what computer games they enjoy the most, they will tell you they are games that provide three-dimensional life-like action. They will also tell you they like to "move the figures around." This is the same advanced technology that has given rise not only to the ability to see the area to be radiated in a three-dimensional context, but also to rotate the image and observe it from different angles. The end result is the ability to make a computer model of the actual prostate gland. The three dimensional aspect of the programming also gives the physician an added advantage of being able to determine the volume of the gland. When I was first diagnosed, all that was told to me was that the transrectal sonogram indicated I had a large prostate. The estimate was about 50cc, plus or minus. It was not until the three-dimensional studies were done with the CT Scan that the volume was ascertained to be 65.3cc. Through this determination it was decided to shrink the gland through the use of hormone therapy before any radiation therapy would be undertaken. Assuming that the size of the gland is not an issue in the therapy to be undertaken, by having this three-dimensional representation of the prostate on the computer, the oncologist is in the best position to determine the approach to be taken to maximize the beam penetration of the prostate.

As stated before the length of the therapy will depend upon whether it is to be the primary form of treatment or as an adjunct to some additional treatment. If it is to be the primary treatment, it is given over a 6 to 8 week period, five days a week. Radiation dosages are given at rates that allow the normal healthy cells to recover somewhat between the daily therapy. The cancerous tissues are not as capable of recovery and they are killed off.

The effectiveness of the three-dimensional radiation therapy is directly related to the dosage of radiation administered to the patient. Because of the conformal nature of the treatment and the ability to have the radiation directed more exactly, higher dosages of radiation can be delivered. The best dosage has not been clearly established at this time, although several studies are underway to ascertain what dosages should be effective with minimal damage to healthy tissue.

There is one other factor to be considered whether to use three-dimensional conformal beam therapy. New equipment and software are constantly being improved, making it easier to narrow the field of the radiation. However, there are some schools of thought that believe that the diagnosis by physicians of the presence of prostate cancer often tends to be too conservative. One of the reasons for re-occurrences of the disease after what appear to be effective and successful treatments (both surgical and radiation) is the presence of microscopic extensions of the cancer outside of the gland. These extensions may not picked up either during surgical pathologic examinations, or by bone scans, MRI's and/or CT Scans when surgery is not utilized. Even negative lymph node biopsies are no guarantee that some microscopic extension from the gland has not taken place. It is therefore important to ask the radiation oncologist: how far out from the "capsule" of the gland will the radiation treat? Early extensions from the gland seem to be no more than 3mm from the capsule. It is for this reason that most radiation plans include a "margin" around the gland for radiation even if there is no definitive proof of the existence of cancer. It is important to ask the extent of margin the radiation oncologist deems sufficient in your situation and why it has been chosen.

Intensity Modulated Radiation Therapy (IMRT)

Intensity Modulated Radiation Therapy, or IMRT, is a relatively new technology. It provides an ability to individualize and alter radiation angles, enabling the radiologist to precisely deliver the doses needed to the area being treated. The IMRT hits the prostate cancer from various angles. The prostate is mapped and imaged prior to the treatment, thus providing the radiologist with a clear picture of the area to be treated. The image created is three-dimensional which is ultimately delivered to the computer system. Prior to any treatment being given a "simulation" is used (called a "phantom"), which enables the physician to determine exactly the doses to be administered during the actual procedure. This therapy allows for a more evenly distributed dosage of radiation. The long-range success of this therapy is still not clear despite years of statistics. Similar radiation systems continue to be developed with the primary aim of reducing the potential for damage to the surrounding tissue, As technology continues to be improved, more directed beam radiation has made it possible to intensify the effect of the treatment

Brachytherapy—Seed Implantation

I had heard of the use of implantation of radioactive materials into human cancers sometime before I investigated its application for prostate cancer. It is not a new concept. Various substances have been utilized over the years, from radioactive gold to various isotopes of iodine. The effectiveness of these treatments over the years has had mixed results. Radiation did kill malignancies, but the placement of the radioactive devices within the tumor inside the body was a hit-and-miss proposition. The further problem with the use of internally planted isotopes was the dosage given off by the implant and the length of time the radiation would remain effective. Without the sophisticated external diagnostic tools we have today, major surgery was often the only way to deliver the radioactive "seeds" or "pellets" to the site of the cancer. Surgery alone carried risk with it, and often the radiation was not effective due to improper placement or low dosage. On the other side of the coin, if the dosage was too great, serious injury to surrounding healthy tissue could and often did occur. With the development of the MRI and CT Scan, as well as new software and advanced computers, the ability to see the "target" without the risk of invasive surgery became a reality. Today, the insertion of a rectal ultrasound probe enables the urologist to get a better visualization of the prostate. These new diagnostic techniques and devices lead to a new radiation therapy for the treatment of prostate cancer—brachytherapy.

As with external beam radiation, there is more than one way to provide this form of radiation therapy: permanent seed implantation and temporary seed implantation. There are also two prime types of radioactive isotopes utilized for the treatment: iodine and palladium seeds. There is still some use of other radioactive isotopes, but the two most common are the ones mentioned. Why different isotopes? Sometimes, the answer depends on the oncologist or urologist's preference, and sometimes on the radiation intensity desired. Palladium has a shorter "half-life." Usually, its radioactive emissions are finished within 10 to 12 weeks after insertion in the body. The dosage tends to be higher than iodine, whose radioactivity may last as long as six months.

An argument exists as to whom is a proper candidate for brachytherapy (you may also see this referred to sometimes as interstitial radiation therapy). The first consideration appears to be the stage of the disease. Most studies indicate that patients with earlier stage tumor-confined prostate cancer are the best candidates for this treatment. Other factors are the Gleason Score, the PSA level and the actual size of the gland. An enlarged prostate due to BPH or genetic factors raises the question as to whether brachytherapy is the right choice. Generally speaking, if the gland is over 45cc, there is a problem as to how effective the implantation of seeds will be. Fortunately, in about 70 percent of men with an enlarged prostate, the gland can be successfully reduced to a size sufficient to use brachytherapy as a therapy. The usual method for gland reduction is to place the patient on hormone therapy for a two to three month period. The hormone therapy is delivered with either a single three-month injection, or with one injection a month. Both approaches are also coupled with daily hormone pills. Some physicians will continue the patient on the hormone therapy for a protracted period during radiation therapy and beyond as an adjunct to the treatment. There are indications that the use of hormone therapy as an adjunct to brachytherapy may be beneficial. There is a growing belief that the effectiveness of the radiation is enhanced when coupled with hormone use.

Similar to the methods utilized for external beam radiation, the use of seed implantation requires knowing exactly where the seeds are to be placed. When this procedure was first utilized in the treatment of prostate cancer, the seeds were placed in the prostate in a free-hand approach. This resulted in too many seeds in some areas of the gland, and "cold spots" in others. The end result was a high degree of failure and a general rejection of this treatment by urologists and oncologists for many years. The development of better diagnostic equipment has virtually eliminated the random placement of the radioactive seeds. Essential to the effective implantation procedure is the use of the CAT Scan before, during, and after the procedure.

The seed implantation is generally performed in a Same Day Surgery setting, although a few medical centers do keep the individual overnight. The procedure is performed under an epidural or spinal anesthesia. Frankly, I never found it essential for me to know what was going on during any medical procedure and I opted for a general anesthesia. In spite of the fact that the radiation oncologist who performed the procedure thought it would be interesting for me to watch the procedure on the monitor, I declined the invitation. The general anesthesia utilized is similar to the rather light anesthesia given for colonoscopies.

I will never again make snide comments about the examination of women and the placing of their feet in stirrups. The procedure for performing the seed implantation is not too dissimilar. You are placed on your back with both your knees bent and your feet elevated. This position provides the ability of providing access to the area where the seeds will ultimately be implanted. The seeds are implanted in the area between the testicles and the anus called the perineum. The needles utilized for the procedure are thin and are preloaded with the particular seeds to be inserted. The seeds themselves are relatively small and are about the size of a small grain of rice. The seeds are placed using a template and are about 10 mm apart. Every effort is made not to place the seeds too close to or in the urethra or rectum. The actual number of the seeds utilized will depend upon the size of the gland. In my situation, I wound up with 117 seeds, which by any definition is a heck of lot of seeds! I joked that with this number I was certain to glow in the dark.

Once the seeds have been placed in this procedure, the physician will perform a post-implant CAT Scan in order to check on the location of the seeds. The urologist will also perform a cystoscopy (insertion of a thin device into the penis) to make certain there are no seeds in the urethra or bladder. As I awoke from the procedure, the physicist was taking a reading of radiation on my lower abdomen and the area of the implant. The Geiger counter did manage a weak clicking sound. I was cautioned that pregnant women, young children, and pets should not sit on your lap for at least six weeks due to the possible radiation leakage from the procedure. Also, I was provided with a strainer and a lead container for the purpose of straining my urine for the next few weeks just in case a seed was to work its way through the urethra. This posed a rather interesting dilemma going to work with my trusty strainer and lead container in my pocket. I often wondered if anyone who saw me in the men's room thought they were standing next to some demented creature. It is remarkable what you learn to put up with when confronted with an illness and its treatment. My normal reserve and potential embarrassment rapidly gave way to a sense that if people didn't understand that was their problem. Fortunately, I did not have this problem, although I did pass a seed through the rectum many months subsequent to the procedure—a fact that mystifies my urologist to this very day!

Most physicians will tell the patient that there is no need for a catheter during the procedure. A catheter is generally put in only for patients with an enlarged prostate. The physician will always do a cystoscopy in order to remove any seeds that are in the bladder or the urethra. My physician inserted a catheter that was left in for three days after the implant was completed. This may have had more to do with the fact that I had the procedure at 2:00PM on a Friday afternoon, than to any other reason! I might add that in general, unless it is an emergency, surgical procedures should not be performed on a Friday afternoon since the weekend creates potential difficulties in securing contact with the physician should the need arise. This is a practical consideration but one which sometimes is overlooked in the rush to undertake treatment. I might note that my physician was and is a unique individual. He was and has been totally available, weekends, at night, whenever needed—a throwback to a more professional period in the practice of medicine.

What was so remarkable about this procedure was the lack of pain or much discomfort after the procedure. There was a sensation of pressure, and when I coughed, there was the feeling that something had transpired. Nothing else. When I sat down, I did feel pressure for a while which I alleviated by sitting on a pillow. My friends insisted on reminding me of the story of the Princess and the Pea and kidded me about being "delicate." I threatened in return to radiate them! After a few days, I became accustomed to the feeling, and the sensation gradually disappeared. The area between my legs was black and blue, including the scrotum. However all of the external evidence of the procedure disappeared after a month or so. I never had any blood in my urine which I had been warned could occur.

The procedure utilizing permanent seeds results in these small radioactive devices remain in the body for life. They are not interactive with the body after the radiation has been expended and cause no problems when left in place. The duration of the radioactivity of the seeds depends upon the isotope used. Palladium-103 has a life expectancy of about 72 days. Iodine-125 has a life expectancy of around 6 months. Which isotope is best for you will depend upon what the radiation oncologist feels is appropriate for your particular condition. From discussions I have had with various physicians, there appears to be a growing preference for the utilization of Palladium 103. The theory is that Palladium gives a greater dosage over a shorter time and may be more effective for more active prostate cancers, i.e. those with higher Gleason Scores.

There is another way to receive brachytherapy treatment—temporary implantation of radioactive seeds. The implantation of radioactive seeds for a temporary period became better known when the Chairman of the Board of Intel Corporation wrote his story for the press. After having researched various approaches to the treatment of prostate cancer, he settled on temporary implantation. The procedure is very similar to the permanent placement of the seeds except that the needles with the radioactive seeds are left in the patient for a day and then removed. This procedure allows for higher dosage to the prostate, but also requires a hospital stay. The procedure is called high-dose rate brachytherapy, (HDR). One of the techniques for the non-permanent radiation of the prostate is the placing of several catheters through the perineal area into the prostate and delivering the radiation through them. The radiation can be delivered on a continual basis over a few days or repeated in a series of sessions. Once the treatment is completed, the catheters are removed. The long-range result of this alternative brachytherapy treatment has not been fully studied, but does provide the ability to opt out of having a life long implant.

The side effects from either form of brachytherapy are minimal in most cases. Sexual potency appears to be initially high, however, long range some studies seem to indicate that potency drops off around the third year after the procedure for about 20 to 40 percent. It is not altogether clear whether this is a function of the age and other physical condition of the patient or due directly to the implant procedure. Urinary urgency and some rectal irritation are more frequent temporary side effects of the implants. This can affect upwards of 25% of patients, but the problem seems to subside in time. From experience, urgency was a major problem for me and started about a week after the procedure. Initially, every hour-and-a-half I had to urinate. This gradually settled into once every two hours, twenty-four hours a day. The condition lasted from June until October when it started to subside. By December, the urinary function was back to normal and sleeping through the night was a decided blessing.

In some studies, rectal ulceration and irritation can occur in 10% to 12% of the men with implants. This problem can be more difficult to cope with and may require changes in diet and other treatment in some cases. Like the problem with urinary urgency, the rectal ulceration appears to be self-correcting in the long run. In my situation, rectal irritation and a need to go to the bathroom after every meal started six months after the procedure and abated after some months. My experience with this rectal problem involved bleeding, a sense of urgency and a mucous discharge. My concern lead to having a colonoscopy that indicated no colon disease or ulcerative condition. The use of rectal suppositories and over the counter preparations such as Metimucil helped and gave the rectum time to heal.

An additional side effect occurred about one year later when all of a sudden I "passed" a seed through the rectum.

What needs to be stressed is that I did not ask all of the right questions when I opted for my treatment. In spite of my research, the extents of the side effects were not as readily apparent as perhaps they could have been. The need to press the physician for a discussion of side effects is very important. Most recently problems with erectile function have also developed. Only now have I discovered that regardless what the literature indicates, impotence may occur sooner then later with virtually all of the treatments. Every day new techniques are being explored to alleviate some of these side effects. As recently as February 2001, Sloan-Kettering Medical Center has been examining the use of drugs when used together with radiation appears to limit damage to surrounding tissue. Increased dosages of Viagra, Levitra, or Cialis appear to address the problem of erectile dysfunction in many men whether treated with surgery or radiation.

Chapter 17

Hormone Therapy

Years past, hormone therapy was used only after the prostate cancer had spread. In affect the hormone was viewed as a holding action hoping to provide an extension of life to men who either had failed prior treatment or were diagnosed with advanced disease. Hormone therapy is employed to block the production of testosterone and androgens primarily by the testes. The use of drugs is in lieu of surgical removal of the testicles. Both accomplish the same result in that they interfere with the manufacture of hormones that tend to nurture and feed the cancer. Hormone therapy may be utilized alone or in combination with any of the other forms of treatment. In my case, I was on hormone therapy for nine months during the 3-D Conformal Radiation and Seed Implantation treatments. In fact, I remained on the hormone therapy for three months beyond the implant procedure. They are given by injection and/or orally. The injected hormone is utilized to stop the production of testosterone by the testes. The daily pills act to block any remaining testosterone from being utilized in the body.

I first became aware of hormones in a high school class and later on in a college course in biology. The extent of my knowledge was fundamental at best. Like most men I had a basic comprehension of the sex hormones to the extent that I knew hormones are part of every human being's makeup and have a direct effect on the growth and general make up of all cellular activity in the body. Some of the strongest hormones are those related to sexuality. I believed that in women there is estrogen and in men it is testosterone. Little did I understand how much more information I would need to comprehend how hormones affect the prostate and cancer growth.

The prostate gland needs more than testosterone in order to grow and perform its function. The process needed for a healthy prostate gland to function requires several activities from various glands of the body. It starts with a gland called the hypothalamus acting as a regulator of secretions from the pituitary gland. The pituitary gland secretions then cause the testes to produce the majority of testosterone. It doesn't end here. The adrenal glands are involved in that they produce about 5% of the testosterone. Additionally, I discovered that the testes also produce estrogen. So much for my simple comprehension of the hormone function of the male body!

It would seem logical if the hormone influence on the prostate could be lessened or totally removed there should be a reduction in the size of the gland and the prostate cancer as well. The issue is how to accomplish this successfully. Testosterone primarily manufactured in the testicles gives rise to an obvious solution, surgical removal of the testicles. This was the basic approach undertaken for many years. This surgery, called an orchidectomy, dramatically reduced the amount of testosterone in the body but often left serious emotional and psychological scars.

Hormone therapy, utilized to accomplish what surgery sought to achieve, is now more prevalent. This therapy tends to alleviate the emotional difficulties associated with surgery. The therapy is divided into two basic types: 1) drugs aimed at switching off the production of testosterone by working on the pituitary gland, and 2) drugs aimed at preventing the body from using the testosterone. Once luteinizing hormone-releasing hormone or LHRH was understood, it led to the development of drugs that switch off the production of testosterone. Lupron, Zoladex, are examples of these drugs. An injection monthly or every three months are given depending upon how the patient responds. The initial effect of the hormonal therapy is that it causes an increase in testosterone levels. This can be a problem if the cancer has already spread. Nonetheless, the overall effect is usually positive for most patients. By also giving anti-androgens or "receptor site blockers" such as Eulexin or Casodex, the physician can prevent this "spike" in testosterone from the hormone injection. These blockers are taken on a daily basis. These drugs perform in the same manner as if the testicles had been surgically removed. It is a form of medical castration without the obvious permanent effects of surgery. Once the drug therapy has been stopped the body will return to the production of testosterone.

The evidence of hormone effectiveness can be seen in the results I encountered while on the drug. My prostate gland shrunk from 65.3cc to approximately 39.cc—40.cc in the initial three-month period. The assumption by my physician was that some of the cancer had been destroyed with this shrinkage as well.

The second arm in the hormone therapy the use of anti-androgens such Casodex in combination with the hormone injection.

For some time, hormone therapy has been given to individuals with advanced prostate cancer with the aim of slowing the growth of the cancer and making the man's life somewhat more comfortable. This palliative hormone treatment does not seek to cure the cancer and is often a viable treatment for older individuals who cannot sustain the rigors of other procedures.

More and more, hormone therapy is being given with a view to assisting in curing the patient of the disease. Considerable studies have started to surface, which discuss the effect of hormone therapy given together with other forms of treatment, such as radiation. These early studies looked at survival rates for men who had advanced but localized prostate cancer and indicated that there was as much as a 20% increase in survival as against those who had only radiation. Because of these early results, many physicians are keeping patients on hormone therapy routinely for periods of nine to twelve months during the course of radiation therapy.

Using myself as an example, I was placed on monthly injections of Lupron in December 1999 along with a daily Casodex pill. I remained on this hormone therapy throughout my subsequent treatment of five weeks of 3-D external conformal beam radiation and Palladium-103 seed implantation. Finally, I was removed from the hormone therapy in September 1999. The hormone treatment lasted a total of nine months, although some urologists are keeping patients on this regime for a twelve-month period. The use of combined therapies such as radiation and hormones is becoming much more common in the treatment of prostate cancer although there is not much long-term evidence of how effective are these combined therapies.

The cost of the hormone therapy is not cheap compared to other treatments. Although cost should not be a factor in life and death struggles, reality must be dealt with in modern society. Some HMO's will not pay for Lupron. The monthly shot can cost upwards of $565.00 per injection and a friend was charged $2000. for the three month injection. He refers to his three-month injection as the "golden needle." The thirty-day supply of the anti-androgen can be as much as $11.00 per daily pill. Monthly costs of $900.00 over a nine to twelve month period are expensive. It is most important that you contact your insurance carrier and ascertain what they will cover for hormone therapy. I was extremely fortunate that my Insurance Plan (not an HMO) picked up the tab for every last nickel of the treatment over the nine-month period, a fact for which I am very grateful.

There are side effects to hormone therapy that gave me a new respect for women who undergo the difficulties of menopause. Not uncommon, I developed hot and cold flashes, a reduced libido, a loss of body hair, and an enlargement of my breasts. The uncontrolled sudden hot sweats were perhaps the most difficult, although they did diminish after a while. Within three months after I was off the hormone therapy, the body hair returned, blessedly brown and not gray, the breasts reduced in size, and the flashes ceased.

Not everyone responds positively to hormone therapy. There are some prostate cancers that are resistant to it. In some situations where the individual has been on hormone therapy for a protracted period, his body has become resistant. In other cases, the prostate cancer is naturally resistant to the hormone therapy for reasons the medical profession does not fully understand. In these situations, science is experimenting with drugs that interfere with a particular protein, Actin. Actin is essential in allowing the cancer cells to break loose from the prostate gland and spread outside the capsule. It accomplishes this feat by dissolving the mechanisms that hold the cancer in place. The newer experimental agents such as TIMP-2; NM 23; and CAI are Actin inhibitors. Other substances have been derived from fruits, vegetables, and sponges all aimed at interfering with the ability of Actin to work. These substances are generally not well known nor understood by most physicians. If you have a hormone-resistant prostate cancer, you may need to seek out a major medical teaching center to secure these alternative treatment options. The Center for Holistic Urology at the Columbia Presbyterian Medical Center in New York City has been investigating several alternative treatments for prostate cancer.

Hormone resistant prostate cancer is a major problem with many men who have been on the hormone therapy for protracted periods of time. New hormones are being tested constantly. Genta Inc. a biopharmaceutical company is in the process of testing a new anti-androgen treatment, which appears to be effective with far fewer side effects, found in the present hormone therapies. However, always remember that even with the development of new treatment options, it takes considerable periods of time to truly assess their effectiveness.

Chapter 18

Monoclonal Antibodies

The more I have sought answers to prostate cancer treatment, the more I was amazed at the breadth of medical research. Medicine is decidedly at the threshold of new treatments for all forms of cancers, including prostate cancer. Not a single day passes without some news release announcing studies and clinical test programs, many of which unfortunately tend to promise much more than usually is delivered. In the early 1970's, science was turning to what seemed to promise a whole new era of cures for all sorts of diseases facilitated through a process known as "genetic engineering." Science was convinced that corrected or perfect cells could be cloned to be exact duplicates of each other in the millions, injected into an individual where they would overtake the defective genes, and cure the individual. It was science fiction come to reality! If cells could be cloned, what of the components of the cells? What of the body's own defense mechanisms—antibodies? From this early research, the development of monoclonal antibodies became a reality.

Monoclonal antibodies, sometimes referred to as MABs, are "disease specific." The antibodies seek out a specific disorder, which is the source of the problem. By targeting them to a specific disease, in theory they should be able to destroy the infection or the cancer wherever it may be found in the body. Further, if the monoclonal antibodies are not capable of actually destroying the bad cell, might they at least locate them? In effect, MABs have a two-prong potential: first, as an actual treatment weapon, and second, as a diagnostic tool. It is these intriguing potentials that have spurred on the development of a separate industry aimed just at the creation of monoclonal antibodies. Imagine an individual diagnosed with prostate cancer, not knowing whether the cancer has escaped the capsule of the gland and spread. The monoclonal antibody can seek out the cancerous cells and either identifies the location of the cells and/or destroys them anywhere in the body. Before you decide that this is the only treatment you need, let's look at what is available in the marketplace and determine whether it suits your needs.

Monoclonal antibodies fall into two distinct categories: those that work by themselves to destroy the cancer or disease, and those that are basically "markers" that will find the cancer or disease but need to be linked with some other agent to do the job. If you can do the job without linking another agent to the antibody, you are ahead of the game. To date, the research results have been mixed. Several companies have marketed and tested various monoclonal antibodies for different diseases with somewhat mixed results. In some cases, remissions of disease were remarkable; yet in others, the results were not as favorable.

The earliest use of monoclonal antibodies in the treatment of prostate cancer started in 1994 and has developed since then. The Roswell Park Cancer Center in Buffalo, New York has received approval for the use of an antibody known as "7E11" (also called "CYT356") for the purpose of diagnosing the location of prostate cancer outside of the gland. This monoclonal antibody is attached to Indium-111 and may provide assistance in finding prostate cancer in the lymph nodes and elsewhere. It is not 100% foolproof. Its market name is ProstaScint. The monoclonal antibody is injected. CAT Scan images are taken at the time of the injection as well as approximately four days thereafter. Some centers utilizing this diagnostic technique also take CAT Scans after the fourth day in order to take advantage of the full effect of the diagnostic treatment. Centers around the nation utilizing this diagnostic approach to prostate cancer are convinced that in the long run, it will prove to be a far better diagnostic technique then either MRI's or CAT Scans. The more you know about the progression of the prostate cancer, the better informed you would be to evaluate the type of treatment that will best suit your needs. There is no doubt that microscopic spread of prostate cancer to the lymph nodes or, to the localized tissue may be difficult to discover by noninvasive examinations. If you have already determined to have radical surgery, the pathologist may or may not pick up microscopic spread, dependent upon what tissue is removed and examined.

There are some problems with ProstaScint that are not unique to many of the monoclonal antibodies being tested in the market today. Monoclonal antibodies work in two fundamental ways. They either penetrate the cell membrane or attack the exterior structure of the cell. If the mechanism is to penetrate the cell, the human body has devised many defenses at the cellular level to prevent such a penetration. In this situation, the risk of not identifying or destroying the cancer is great, and the potential of lingering disease is a major risk.

Major medical centers such as Yale New Haven, The Lahey Clinic, and Johns Hopkins have been investigating various forms of monoclonal antibodies as possible treatments instead of use only for diagnostic purposes. One issue that no one has an answer to at present is whether all prostate cancers are sufficiently similar so that a single monoclonal antibody would be effective against all of them. It is very likely that every patient might need to have unique monoclonal antibodies created for their own needs.

In spite of the uncertainty of the future direction of this form of diagnostic treatment, it is an additional avenue that the prostate cancer patient needs to be aware of in order to make informed and intelligent decisions about treatment. In an era where mankind has cloned sheep, monkeys, and, most recently in Japan, actual animal organs, monoclonal antibodies are not to be dismissed. Questions need to be raised with the treating physician as to the benefit of availing yourself of test programs utilizing monoclonal antibodies for diagnosis and clinical treatment of your prostate cancer.

Aligned with the development of MABs has been the search for a viable vaccine that would be effective against cancer. The theory is simple; get the body to use its own immune system to fight the disease. If the immune system could mobilize the T-Cells in the body to attack the cancer could a vaccine be far behind? John Hopkins Medical Center has been experimenting with a procedure where they take the malignant tumor out of the patient. The tumor is treated with radiation to prevent the cells from dividing. A new gene is added to the cells and injected back into the patient. This new gene (GM-CSF) attacks the surface of the cancer cells cutting up a chemical. In turn the T-Cells attack the cut up pieces of the tumor and continue to go after all similar cancer receptors. It all sounds like science fiction or something out of horror movie, but it appears to hold promise. In some patients who have undergone this treatment, their PSA levels have dropped more than 50%. Does the drop in PSA indicate the cancer is no longer aggressive? Is this vaccine approach the cure of the future? It is too early to know and the numbers of patients treated are too small from which to derive good statistical data. I personally am certain that I would not have opted for this treatment due to the lack of long-term proof of its effectiveness.

Chapter 19

Holistic—The Herbal Approach

You cannot turn on a radio or watch television without seeing advertisements for various herbal remedies, vitamins and minerals. We live in an era of Health Food Stores and the search for miracle cures through nature. For years-traditional medicine looked askance at any suggestion that there might be alternative approaches to the treatment and cure for diseases. In recent times, however, studies have eroded the attitudes of traditional medical practitioners and have discovered that there are natural herbal supplements that do have healing properties. More and more in the treatment of prostate cancer, diet and herbal supplements appear to provide prevention as well as control of prostate diseases, including prostate cancer. More physicians are not only looking at "complementary" treatments but are actively prescribing them to their patients. As in other areas of prostate treatment, time is needed to provide reasonable validation of any treatment, and the jury is still out on the long-range effectiveness of these therapies. However, as my sainted mother used to say about chicken soup, "it may not help, but it can't hurt." Some of the holistic treatments have been around for several years in other countries and do appear to have positive effects on prostate conditions. A word of caution is needed. Even holistic remedies that have existed for centuries can carry with them serious risks that can be discovered only after careful clinical study. Of greater concern is the effect of holistic medications with prescription drugs. Even drinking grapefruit juice while ingesting holistic medication can be a deadly combination.

Not too many years ago, I remember asking a friend of mine, a Professor of Medicine at a major New York City University medical school and hospital, about the role of complementary medical treatment for diseases. I specifically raised the issue about the diet factor as a cause of cancer and similar disorders. For thirty minutes I listened to a lecture from my friend about "quacks," "phony holistic healers," "overstated promises of miracle food cures," and why "people get taken down the fool's path by listening to such garbage." I did get an admission that low fat diets were helpful in some cases in lowering high cholesterol levels. There was also an admission from the Professor that high fiber diets were in fact helpful in lowering the risk of colorectal problems, including cancer. However, beyond the already accepted medical pronouncements, no quarter was given to any other approach to the treatment of disease, especially cancers. This was not a unique experience. Even where younger physicians might be open to possible advantages of holistic treatment, it was not broadly embraced. It appeared that modern medicine had completely forgotten about the evolution of herbal and natural remedies. This has been compounded by the fact that the latter half of the Twentieth Century has been the era of chemically compounded medicines, which in the minds of the medical profession was far superior to anything nature had to offer.

The picture has started to change dramatically. The use of holistic treatment for prostate cancer has become a hot topic. What has precipitated this change? First, is the realization that there is still much to learn about the causes of prostate cancer and why it is much more common in Western than in Asian society? Second, is the investigation into differences in dietary practices in various parts of the world and how they appear to affect not only the development of not only prostate cancer but other disorders as well. Third, is a better understanding of the workings of cellular structures of the human body and the various influences on them. Putting together all of these factors has forced a rethinking of traditional medical practices.

The willingness to investigate nontraditional methods of treating disease has not been limited to inquisitive patients and single practitioners. Major institutions such as Memorial-Sloan Kettering Cancer Center and Columbia-Presbyterian Medical Center are viewing the patient in holistic terms. The Director of the Prostate Diagnostic Center at Memorial-Sloan Kettering has been vocal in pointing to the effectiveness of complimentary approaches to prostate cancer treatment. Dr. Aaron Katz at Columbia-Presbyterian headed up The Center for Holistic Urology with a dedicated view of examining the effect of herbal and vitamin therapy in the treatment of prostate cancer. Some of the treatments being investigated have long histories in Asian medical practices. The FDA has not been happy with some of the holistic approaches to prostate cancer treatment, specifically because of serious side effects, but also due to the inability to secure consistent contents of some of the formulas used. Some of the holistic remedies have not been thoroughly tested through the use of "double-blind" studies. It must be understood that merely because an herb or combination of herbs has been utilized for several years does not indicate that they are an effective treatment for the disease.

Assisting this willingness to investigate new holistic treatments has been investigation in the role of anti-oxidants in protection of cellular structure. It became apparent that certain vitamins, minerals, and other substances were successful in protecting the human body from the damage caused by the body's creation of free radicals. Free radicals can damage the DNA of the cell and give rise to cancerous conditions.

Some of the holistic products used as prostate treatments have been around for several years. Many were used first in Europe and Asia with varying degrees of success. Considerable data has been gathered over the years supporting several herbal remedies.

Saw Palmetto made from berries has been tested extensively and found to be beneficial in reducing the BPH symptoms in many men. It also has been shown to shrink the prostate and be a diuretic in nature. Often, Saw Palmetto is combined with zinc, which appears to be supportive of proper prostate function. The actual effect of either Saw Palmetto or zinc in fighting prostate cancer is still not proven. Nonetheless, the ability of Saw Palmetto to shrink the gland would appear to have some effect on the growth of the cancer within the gland. More testing is needed and is under way to determine the extent to which this herb may slow or even aid in the cure of prostate cancer.

The common tomato and tomato products have been in the press recently. Tomato products appear to present an interesting new development in the area of holistic substances utilized in fighting of prostate cancer. Lycopene is the substance that gives the tomato its red color. Lycopene appears to have a very positive effect on prostate health and may actually destroy the prostate cancer. Individuals with high levels of tomato ingestion, especially through processed tomato products such as sauces, catsup, juice, and soup, are less likely to experience prostate cancer.

Lycopene also appears to reduce the cancer in the prostate once it has been detected. More importantly, Lycopene seems to slow the progression of prostate cancer and prolongs the remission of the disease. As is the case with most of the holistic herbal treatments, Lycopene is available over the counter without prescription. Once again, time will be the ultimate proof of whether these claims are a "flash in the pan" or hold out hope for more important applications in the fight against prostate cancer.

For years, the Chinese touted green tea as a cure for cancer and several other disorders. Scientists have recently confirmed the anti-oxidant properties in green tea and its ability to limit certain enzymes responsible for cancer tumors. Green tea also limits the development of the necessary blood supply to tumors. This is a major area of cancer research. If the blood supply to tumors can be reduced or cut off, the tumor dies. Most cancer tumors develop sources of blood supply for the purpose of feeding the cells. If green tea can limit the development of these blood supplies the effect is self-evident!

The recommended consumption is three cups of green tea per day. No treatment is free of side effects. The green tea does contain caffeine, which must be taken into account if you have a reaction to caffeine. There is decaffeinated green tea in the stores. Unfortunately, I have been unable to determine whether the process of decaffeinating adversely effects the potency of the tea. I have seen recent reports that state all teas are potent anti-oxidants, but green tea is the best. I like tea but I am not certain how many cups a day are required. My Chinese friends tell me they drink seven to ten cups a day. My side effect with all teas is my need to be near a bathroom after a third cup!

Vitamins, A, C, E, and selenium have been investigated as playing a role as potential cancer preventers. Their role in regressing or killing existent cancers is not clear. In spite of uncertainties connecting prostate cancer prevention with vitamins, institutions such as Sloan Kettering advocates Vitamin E and a low saturated fat diet to prevent prostate cancer. As stated earlier, the international SELECT study is specifically studying the effect of Vitamin E and selenium as possible prostate cancer preventers. Unfortunately this is a twelve-year study which doesn't help much if you have already been diagnosed with the disease.

Two other holistic treatments have been shown to have a direct impact on prostate cancer. Soybeans possess ingredients that kill prostate cancer cells. Isoflavone is the element that affects the growth of the cancer cells. In Asian societies such as Okinawa, there is a direct correlation between low prostate cancer levels and the ingestion of soy products. Once the Okinawan moves to the West, his risk of prostate cancer rises to the level of the Western society. Laboratory tests indicate that it is the Isoflavone and enzymes in the soybean that appear to reduce the prostate cancer. Unfortunately, over the past few months, some troubling data has come to the attention of researchers. The studies state soy and soy products may have a serious side effect resulting in the shrinkage of brain tissue. Although this recent concern is still under study, it illustrates the problem in accepting without careful study even the common food substances that initially appear to offer hope in the treatment of diseases.

In the last few years, a combination of eight holistic elements has appeared on the market under the commercial label, PC-SPES. The use of PC-SPES has been shown to lower the serum levels of PSA dramatically in-patients with prostate cancer, with out further progression of the disease. Levels of testosterone were markedly reduced. However, there were potential serious side effects to the use of this product. Some men developed blood clots in the legs. Others developed side effects similar to those when using hormones, including breast soreness, hot flashes, and sexual dysfunction.

The use of holistic treatment for prostate cancer is still very much in its infancy. The effect of the interaction of taking several holistic treatments needs to be understood. The FDA has been critical of PC-SPES for the reasons set forth above and has banned its use. Recently a class-action law suit was commenced against the manufacturer of the commonly sold brand of PC SPES due to the high rate of serious side effects caused by this product.

Although these doubts do exist, I did start taking Saw Palmetto three times a day for a total of six pills or 3000mg prior to the diagnosis of my prostate cancer. After my diagnosis and the termination of all medical therapies, I also started taking 800mg of Vitamin E; 100mg of Selenium; 15mg of Lycopene; and 600mg of Beta Sito Sterol. Beta Sito Sterol is a substance advertised as aiding in urinary control by shrinking the prostate. Have any of these holistic treatments helped to prevent a return of my prostate cancer or control any cancer that is still present? I do not have the answer and may never know. As the old saying goes when asking whether chicken soup really does any good, "it may not do any good, but it can't hurt!"

What is clear is that diet does play an important role in the scheme of things. There is more evidence that low fat diet and a greater intake of fruits and vegetables lowers the risk of prostate and other cancers in the body.

Chapter 20

Wait and Watch

Probably the most controversial therapy is no therapy at all. This involves doing nothing but waiting, and observing the prostate cancer. For years, there has been a small but very vocal school of medical thought that has questioned the wisdom of undertaking more traditional therapies immediately. Part of the philosophy in waiting and watching has to do with the age of the man diagnosed with prostate cancer. For men over seventy years of age, the statistical odds seem to favor no treatment—especially if the cancer is capsule confined and the Gleason Score is low. The theory is that prostate cancer is a slow growing disease and is symptom free in its early stages. While prostate cancer does kill, the older individual will probably die of some other disorder before it reaches the critical stage.

There are truths to this approach, however. To the extent that the patient can live with the thought of an untreated cancer in his body, he may decide that no treatment is acceptable. The real problem is that if a man is in his seventies and in good health otherwise, his life expectancy may be far longer then the actuary table sets forth. Further, there are several unknown factors pertaining to prostate cancer. Sloan Kettering Memorial Hospital has recently indicated that there appear to be two distinct forms of prostate cancer. Whether these forms grow at different rates or respond to therapies differently is not clear. It would be a tragedy to find out too late that your prostate cancer was of the type that was far more virulent and needed some form of medical intervention to prevent a more rapid progression. There may be additional reasons to wait and watch. The physical condition of the patient may be such that more traditional therapies are not feasible. Last, but certainly not least, many men who look at the potential side effects of the more traditional therapies elect to do nothing more than to have their prostate cancers observed closely recognizing that prostate cancer is relatively slow growing.

"Wait and watch" proponents point to the most troubling of all factors; several studies seem to indicate that regardless of what treatment is undertaken, the potential of reoccurrence may be the same for individuals with low PSA levels, Gleason Scores and capsule confined cancers. Even with more aggressive treatment, statistics seem to be somewhat supportive of the fact that in the long run, it may not matter what the patient undertakes to utilize as the basis of therapy. This is a sobering thought to say the least.

There is the other side of the coin within the medical community, which states that regardless of the age of the patient, some form of affirmative treatment is always required, essential, and beneficial. While this attitude may make sense assuming the man is vital, vibrant, and young in spite of his age, there are problems in undertaking treatments that destroy or lessen the quality of life of an older man with no long term benefit to be secured. With the exception of "wait and watch" approaches to prostate cancer, all of the other treatments will carry with them some potential for side effects and discomfort. As recent articles in the New England Journal of Medicine indicate, if there is validity to relating the rapid rise in PSA levels in the year proceeding diagnosis, "Wait and Watch" may not be a sound approach to dealing with the disease.

As I indicated earlier with older men, the approach to watch and wait tends to become an option that is appealing to many men of all ages. I have a friend in his mid eighties who is a retired physician. He is presently on dialysis and has some other medical problems. He has indicated to me that his PSA is rising although he has no other symptoms. When questioned what he intends to do about his rising PSA, he has consistently indicated that he will merely watch and wait and see if he develops any other symptoms. If he were in relatively perfect health, watching and waiting for him would still probably be his choice based upon his age as the most telling factor. This does not mean that his decision is either right or wrong; rather, it is the one that makes sense for him.

As for the younger man such as myself, although not cancer-phobic, the prospect of waiting and watching the prostate cancer was never an option—especially in the light of a rising PSA and a moderate range Gleason Score. In retrospect, however, I ask myself: if my prostate cancer is slow growing and I had no symptoms of any prostate problem, would I have the courage to sit back and do nothing but observe the progression of my disease, even if I were older? I am not certain that I could have undertaken that course of action.

Perhaps most basic to the "wait and watch" philosophy is whether there is a point in time when no treatment is the best treatment. Assuming that at some subsequent point in time it appears that the cancer is becoming more aggressive, is that the time when treatment should be undertaken? There are some studies under way at the Memorial Sloan Kettering Medical Center that would lead one to believe that there may be different forms of prostate cancer. If this theory proves to be correct the next obvious issue will be whether they act differently and whether different approaches to treatment of the prostate cancer may be required. I have heard many physicians state that they are not certain that prostate cancer needs to be treated if as they suspect the disease is a natural occurrence of male aging. If these suppositions are correct then prostate cancer may have a more benign long-term implication for most men.

Watching and waiting may not involve doing "nothing." Several studies have combined watching and waiting with a change to a low fat vegetarian diet coupled with stress management and exercise. At present there is a California study assessing the effect of vegetarian diets along with programmed exercise and stress management programs on men with prostate cancer. The participants in this study have all been diagnosed with prostate cancer and have opted to follow this regimen along with the above changes in their life styles. The program has been in existence for a short period of time and therefore is far too early to known if there is a basis to this modified approach.

Presently, once prostate cancer has spread there are few treatments available which seem to be effective in reversing the progress of the disease. With this as a potential long-term risk, the decision to watch and wait must be undertaken with the utmost thought.

Reported in the May 2005 issue of The New England Journal of Medicine was a new study indicating that in younger men, "watching and waiting" did not fare as well as those undergoing surgery. The study did not compare surgery however to any other form of treatment.

Recent studies reported in February 2006 have cast serious doubts on whether it is advisable to merely watch and wait to see what develops once prostate cancer has been diagnosed. For several years the attitude in the medical community was not to initiate any therapy with older men diagnosed with the disease. The feeling was that in most cases men over 70 would die with the disease rather than from it. As men are living longer productive lives, this philosophy has come into serious question. The new studies indicate that some form of treatment is far better for the man than doing nothing. Recognize that to watch and wait is ultimately an individual decision.

Chapter 21

What Is The Right Treatment For You?

I have not set forth every treatment or variations in the previous discussion. There are as many different approaches as there are physicians and researchers in the field of prostate cancer. Do yourself a favor and repeat— "Knowledge is power!" The more you understand the nature of prostate cancer, the better equipped you are to make the intelligent treatment choices. I came to realize that each urologist, radiologist, and oncologist with whom I discussed my condition had his or her own treatment approach. Each physician believes his or her approach is the correct one. This is not stated as a criticism. People have comfort levels with what they know. When you have dealt with a problem for several years, change is difficult. New treatments for prostate cancer carry risks with them. There is the risk of not knowing all of the ramifications of the new treatment. What are the side effects? What is the long-range prognosis if I follow a particular treatment? Unfortunately, bad results may not only give rise to a reoccurrence of the prostate cancer, but with it, the potential risk of litigation for the physician especially if the patient has been told a particular treatment will cure the cancer. If you seek a nonsurgical option, be certain it is a recognized and well-established procedure. If a urologist is treating you who is comfortable only in performing a prostatectomy, then you need to know what you want. As a close physician friend of mine likes to state, "surgeons are trained to cut!"

Second opinions are absolutely essential if you are to arrive at the right treatment for you. Unlike other illnesses, prostate cancer poses a different requirement for second opinions. With prostate cancer, you need to contact different "types" of physicians. Not only do you need to talk to the urologist/surgeon, but also to oncologists and radiologists. I discovered that the younger the physician the greater the flexibility in presenting treatment options. Seek out younger physicians who may have been trained in more current techniques. The younger physicians I questioned were realistic and not afraid to respond to my pointed questions. Do not be panicked into making rash decisions. With prostate cancer, you have a reasonable amount of time to engage in shopping around for different viewpoints.

How do you secure physicians who will provide you with second opinions? In addition to referral to medical societies in the local area, word of mouth from friends can be very helpful. With the increase in the numbers of men diagnosed with prostate cancer, it is amazing how many of my friends have the disease. Although everyone approaches illness differently, friends are a good starting point for referrals. Since writing this book no fewer than five acquaintances have been diagnosed with prostate cancer. Each one has come to me for information and my experiences. Another good source for second opinions is to ask the physician who has diagnosed your condition. I was pleasantly surprised at the willingness of physician that originally diagnosed me to provide names of other specialists. A word of caution—do not rely on these inputs alone. In larger cities where there may be several major medical centers, call up the hospitals and ask for referrals. In less accessible locales, find out where the nearest major center may be and take a trip—it will be worth it in the long run!

The most productive way to ascertain the best treatment is to ask pointed and detailed questions. In some situations these questions lend themselves to being asked even before you have been diagnosed. I have put together the following series of questions. I asked all of them!

These questions should provide a basis in helping you decide your right treatment. In any event whatever treatment you determine suits your needs, always remember: once you have decided upon a treatment, never look back and regret what treatment options you have chosen.

1. How often do I need to have my PSA taken?

2. If the PSA levels swing widely, does this automatically mean I may have prostate cancer?

3. When should a biopsy be performed? Where will the biopsy be performed and who will actually do the procedure? What does the procedure entail? Are there side effects, pain, or any potential dangers to having the procedure? How many core samples will be taken of the prostate during the procedure?

Keep in mind that if your physician has informed you that your prostate is enlarged, more core biopsy samples may be required. Question the physician carefully whether he or she believes the numbers of biopsy samples are adequate for the size of the gland.

4. Can I have both BPH and prostate cancer and does one affect the treatment of the other?

5. If the biopsy is positive, what stage prostate cancer do I have?

6. How did you decide the stage of my prostate cancer?

7. What was my Gleason Score and how was it determined?

8. May I please have the pathology slides of the biopsy so I can have another pathologist read them?

9. What treatments have you utilized for the stage, Gleason Score, and PSA levels with which I have been diagnosed?

10. What have been the results you have achieved long range with the treatments you have utilized?

11. Are there other treatment options available than the ones you utilize?

12. Do you have the names of physicians and/or medical centers utilizing other treatment options?

13. Do you recommend a particular treatment for my form of prostate cancer? How familiar are you with this treatment? How long have you performed this treatment with other patients having similar stages of the prostate cancer?

14. How often will I need these treatments?

15. Over what period of time will these treatments be given?

16. How urgent is it that I commence these treatments if I elect to use the one you recommend?

17. If I have questions during the treatment, who will provide the answers?

18. Who will be the physician following up after I have completed my course of treatment?

19. How uncomfortable will the treatment be?

20. Will I be able to continue with my usual life patterns during the treatment?

21. Is there a recuperation period after the end of the treatment? Approximately how long will this period be?

22. Do you see a cure or control of my prostate cancer as the goal for the treatment you recommend?

This question must be faced head on. Any physician, who will tell you that once undertaken, a certain form of treatment will "cure" the prostate cancer should be immediately replaced. The reality, as uncomfortable as it may be, is that no physician can tell you that a particular treatment is a "cure," in good conscience. Early detection is having a profound impact on survival rates for prostate cancer sufferers. Indeed, it would appear that the long-term rates of success might be as high as 70%. Only time can tell how well the treatment has attacked the prostate cancer. The time frame we are talking about is measured in terms of ten to fifteen years. I have been extremely troubled by the media which in its' ignorance constantly indicates in reports about prostate cancer, that if caught early and the prostate is removed, you are cured. Further, even lay spokespersons that have had the surgical removal of their prostate also talk about being cured. Prostate cancer plays out over a long period of time. In most cases, time will be the ultimate judge of whether the procedure you have undertaken has in fact stopped the cancer and its progression.

23. From your experience and looking at my diagnosis, how realistic are the chances for long term survival?

24. What are the side effects of this treatment?

I was as guilty as most men in not pressing this particular question. Every form of treatment for prostate cancer has potential side effects. The statistics for the type of side effect you may develop does not guaranty you will or will not get them. However, if for example the potential for impotence for men receiving a treatment is 84%, you need to clearly understand that your risk for impotence with that treatment will be almost a statistical certainty. If your sex life is an important "quality of life" issue this must be known prior to the selection of the treatment.

25. Are these side effects temporary or permanent?

Temporary or permanent is very relative term. A temporary side effect that lasts up to two years is pretty close to "permanent" to my thinking. My urge incontinence lasted from June through until December. Those six months felt like a lifetime. Recognize also that no physician can promise that any side effect will in fact disappear. With many treatments, the physician can only provide a range of weeks or months. If you are lucky, then you have no side effects. Otherwise they must be measured by your ability to cope.

26. If these side effects are permanent, how badly will they impact on my quality of life?

27. If these side effects are temporary, how long do you expect them to last and how will it affect my quality of life during the duration of them?

28. Are there any known treatments to alleviate the impact of the side effects?

Some side effects such as impotence may be relieved through the use of new medicines such as Viagra. If medications do not work, surgical intervention may be required. Find out the statistics!

29. When will I know whether the treatment is effective?

30. Will you inform me of new developments that may either augment or replace the treatment I am undergoing?

31. Once the treatments are over, how often should I check my PSA level?

With procedures other than surgery, your PSA may be checked every three months for up to a year or two then once every six months for a year then once a year. Even with surgery, checking the PSA is important to ascertain if all of the cancer has been removed. Every physician has a slightly different approach to the post treatment taking of the PSA test.

32. What further treatments are available to me if this treatment fails?

No one likes to approach a serious illness on a negative footing. It may be helpful to find out what follow up treatment is available in the event the initial procedure is unsuccessful. After radiation (external or seed implantation) surgery may no longer be an option. You need to understand before you undertake treatment what I like to call "the potential phase two of the disease."

33. What are the costs of this treatment compared to other treatments available? Do you know whether insurance will cover them?

The issue of pressing what side effects you may experience is extremely important. This becomes the core of the "quality of life issue." Physicians tend to underplay the side effects. They cannot be totally blamed for this lapse. Patients tend to be reluctant to tell their physicians the truth especially when the side effect concerns impotence. The macho image has made it very difficult for many men to be open about pain, incontinence and sexual dysfunction. There is enough evidence however that certain procedures may well cause side effects that can be very disconcerting. Physicians often throw about statistics as if to lessen concerns. Press the physician directly as to what has been the physicians' particular experience with the treatments he or she has utilized. Most important forget your macho image and be up front about what would upset your quality of life if it were to occur.

These questions are certainly not all inclusive. Yet they do provide a basis for helping you evaluate the physician as well as giving you a clearer understanding of what may be the most acceptable treatment for your needs and desires. As I have indicated earlier in the book, the more you know about the disease and the options available, the better equipped you will be to determine the path that makes you the most comfortable. Do not be afraid to take a written list of these questions with you when you are examined. Also take a friend, a spouse, a significant other in order to make certain the answers you are given are remembered correctly. If necessary write down the answers the physician gives.

If the physician with whom you are speaking does not have the time or the inclination to respond to your questions, find another physician. Remember that it is your body and your choices. You are entitled to the answers to your concerns.

PART III

RECURRENCE CONSIDERATIONS

Chapter 22

Diagnosis

One of the realties of prostate cancer appears to be the fact that in many situations it makes little difference what treatment is undertaken, since the possibility of reoccurrence of the disease may be a statistical reality in many cases. What is becoming apparent concerning prostate cancer is that some forms of this disease may be more aggressive then others and may have already spread beyond the gland at the time when initial treatment is undertaken. To make matters worse, in some instances there may be no observable evidence that the cancer has spread at the time of diagnosis. Microscopic disease is often not detectable even when surgery has been the course of treatment undertaken. On occasion when the pelvic lymph node has not been removed and examined, there may be evidence of a spread to the node that goes undetected. Local spread may also be at the microscopic level and not easily discernible by the surgeon. In cases where other treatment options have been undertaken, the pelvic lymph node would not be removed and an MRI or CAT Scan might not indicate a low level of spread. PET Scans although tending to detect disease spread better than MRI or CAT Scans is extremely expensive and in some situations may not be covered by insurance. Even if there has been a spread of the prostate cancer, the reality is that the spread may not be rapid and may not reach discernable levels for many months or even years.

With greater publicity and awareness on the part of the general community, men are being diagnosed early in the progression of the disease. Many men have no tumors that are susceptible of being felt by a DRE. In theory, this would lead most to believe that treatment at these early stages would present the greatest possibility of a "cure." Yet there are troubling indications that other factors, such as significant rising PSA levels prior to diagnosis, may correlate to future reoccurrence or even evidence of an existent spread of the disease. The conclusion reached in recent published clinical studies is indeed very sobering. Men, who had a rise of 2.0ng in their PSA per year prior to their diagnosis and then underwent radical surgery or some other form of treatment, had a reoccurrence within seven years from diagnosis. It must be remembered, however, that these are statistics and not guaranteed forecasts.

The first and most important question that needs to be answered concerns when the cancer has returned. Historically, a rising PSA level will indicate that there is something going on that need to be investigated.

Individuals who have had other forms of radiation therapy for the treatment of their prostate cancer will have some PSA reading after treatment has ended. Here again rising levels of PSA will be an indicator of changes in the system. Not every rise in PSA levels will be a sign of a reoccurrence. Those men who have had non-surgical treatment may find that their prostate glands have started to enlarge, indicating perhaps a BPH condition. There may be infections or irritations of the prostate.

In 2001 studies conducted at Duke University and Johns Hopkins Medical Center, the use of a diagnostic imaging agent entitled "ProstaScint" appeared to improve the ability to more effectively diagnose the presence of recurrent prostate cancer as well its location and extent. ProstaScint is a monoclonal antibody that targets a particular membrane found on prostate cancer cells. Obviously, the ability to quickly find and locate the recurrent cancer is extremely helpful in determining what treatment should be undertaken.

Other methods of detection of recurrent disease include CT Scan, MRI and X-Ray. On occasion, ultrasound may also indicate the presence of recurrent disease. The best advice is to continue to have routine urologic examinations. In the event that you experience unusual symptoms such as changes in urinary flow rates; more frequency of urination; pains in the back; pelvic region; thighs, see your urologist as soon as possible. In all probability there is nothing wrong, but as my mother was often heard to say: "Better safe then sorry!"

Chapter 23

Treatment Options

Having ascertained that the prostate cancer has returned, you are now faced with some of the same dilemmas that confronted you when you were originally diagnosed with the disease. There are some differences, however, when the disease reoccurs. Depending upon the initial treatment you had, there may be limitations on subsequent options available to you. When the First Edition of this book was written, the limitations were greater then today. New techniques have created more options and greater understanding of how to deal with reoccurring disease. Recurrence will often dictate what treatment to undergo based simply upon the extent of the spread of the disease and the general physical condition of the individual. Often the disease has spread locally in the general pelvic region and not beyond into the bones of the back, thighs or ribs. The disease may not have spread to the pelvic lymph nodes or to the distant lymph nodes of other portions of the body. The age of the man may also be a factor in determining what treatment should be undertaken. Obviously, an older man in his eighties may not desire to undergo extensive therapy nor may it be advisable if the disease is still localized in the pelvic region and not causing discomfort. All of these factors become as much a part of the decision process as when the prostate cancer was first diagnosed in the individual. Each man must also decide for himself the extent and type of treatment he is willing to undergo if the disease does reoccur.

Cryosurgery

Although there are some physicians who disagree, if a man has had his prostate cancer treated primarily through the use of radiation, additional radiation is often not a choice for reoccurrence. Cryosurgery has become more appealing as a subsequent treatment for localized reoccurring prostate cancer. New techniques that utilize thermocoupiers that protect the surrounding tissue have removed much of the potential damage to good tissue that occurred in the past.

Through the use of ultrasound to guide the physician, precise location of the treatment can be achieved. The side effects are, however, not to be overlooked and must be evaluated. There is an overwhelming chance that you will become impotent through the use of cryosurgery. There is also the risk of incontinence, rectal injury and some pelvic discomfort. The procedure is performed as an out patient same-day surgery for most men, with an overnight stay for a small minority.

As more time passes, cryosurgery is also taking on greater significance as a primary treatment for the disease as indicated early on in this book.

What if the prostate cancer is not localized in the pelvic region? Obviously in such a circumstance while cryosurgery may address the localized situation it will not be effective systemically and other treatments may be required in addition to treating the localized spread of the disease.

Hormone Treatment

Hormone treatment for reoccurring prostate cancer has been utilized for several years. Leuprolide and like drugs are administered in the attempt to slow down the spread of the disease. The goal is the same as when given to men when they are first diagnosed with the disease. The initial advantage is that the hormone has a systemic affect on the body. In the event that the cancer has spread beyond the pelvic region, the hormone can shut down up to 95% of testosterone production in the body. Leuprolide is the usual hormone given for the treatment or recurring prostate cancer.

Sometimes different hormone approaches may be tried in an attempt to chemically have the same effect as the removal of the testes. These hormones, however, do not seem to be as effective as Leuprolide.

Hormone therapy requires constant blood tests to measure the level of the hormone in the system together with appropriate Cat Scans to ascertain the status of the disease.

The down-side to hormone treatment is that it sometimes does not work even over the short haul. In such cases other treatments have to be undertaken. A rather traditional approach has been to surgically remove the testes. When the hormone therapy does work, the patient may become resistant to the effect of the hormone after some time has elapsed. Clearly the older the patient, the more likely that with any luck, the patient on hormone therapy will die with prostate cancer rather than from prostate cancer!

Chemotherapy

The early use of chemotherapy treatment with recurring prostate cancer was not promising. As late as the last decade most physicians did not consider chemotherapy as a serious option to the treatment of recurring prostate cancer.

Steriods had been tried but with marginal success until some benefits were shown by combining the steroids with a drug called mitoxantrone. This combination resulted in reductions of pain and as a result the ability to continue life with some degree of quality. The problem with a considerable number of recurring prostate cancers is the tendency of the disease to spread to the bones of the thighs and back. Bone disease can be extremely debilitating and painful. Therefore, any treatment that can alleviate the pain will naturally improve one's quality of life. Although steroid in combination with other drugs is still utilized, the reality of this treatment is that its apparent effect is marginal at best, and only seems to work in about a third of patients who undertake this form of combined drug therapy.

More recently new chemotherapies have been investigated. Drugs such as docetaxel [also known as "Taxotere"], paclitaxel and estranmustine have all been studied in various combinations as well as alone. The results in these studies appear more promising than the earlier chemotherapies in that almost half of the men on these treatments appear to positively respond to them. In June 2004, at the meeting of the American Society of Clinical Oncology, much attention was given to the expanded use of docetaxel as chemotherapy for later stage recurring prostate cancer. Perhaps what is as interesting is that docetaxel had previously been approved for treating breast cancers.As more break-throughs occur in the treatment of breat cancer, there is hope that more of the breast cancer drugs may have a beneficial impact on advanced prostate cancer.

With the increased study of biogenetic factors in the general field of cancer research, agents that inhibit growth of cells have also been looked to as potential additional treatments for recurring prostate cancer.

New drugs are coming out at an increasing rate. Exisulind was experimented with in 2001 under the trade name Apotosyn, and appeared in a small study to delay the progression of the disease.

Radiation

If the primary treatment received was not radiation therapy, such as removal of the prostate, hormone treatment, cryosurgery, waiting and watching, then various forms of radiation are still available to be utilized to attack the recurring prostate cancer. This encompasses external as well as internal radiation therapies. For a full description of the types of radiation therapy that could be undertaken, please refer back to those sections of Chapter 15 that discuss the forms of radiation available.

Vaccine

There have been attempts to create a form of vaccine to treat men whose prostate cancer has returned. In a report publicized in February 2005, in a very small test of 127 men treated with a vaccine called "Provenge," there appears to be some marginal success. Utilizing a protein found in most prostate cancers, and modified to each individual, the vaccine uses the immune cells from each man and is given in the form of three treatments over a month. Men treated with vaccine survived about four and a half months longer than those individuals who had been given a placebo. What is perhaps more significant is that after three years, a third of the men who had received the vaccine were still alive, while only 10 percent of the men who received the placebo were still living.

Clearly, it is still too early to know the significance of vaccine treatment for recurring prostate cancer. However, what this study does illustrate is that the use of an individual's own immune system may hold a key to fighting off the disease after it has already taken hold, rather than the usual use of vaccines to prevent the disease from occurring in the first place.

Chapter 24

What To Do If The Cancer Returns

There are no simple answers to the question raised by the Chapter heading.

First: There must be a determination as to where the cancer has spread.

Second: You must be knowledgeable about the primary treatment you underwent when the prostate cancer was first diagnosed.

Third: You must also be aware that each available therapy carries with it certain potential side effects that can either be of short duration or permanent.

In very blunt terms, if the disease has spread well beyond the local pelvic region into many distant parts of your body, you must make a decision concerning whether you want to undergo extensive treatments that may have limited effect in slowing the progression of the disease (with all of the potential additional discomfort associated with the therapy), or to merely be made as pain free and comfortable as possible. I know I have always expressed my strong convictions if this situation would confront me. Each man needs to address not only the realities of this when if occurs, but also consider it in the context of his ethical, moral and religious beliefs.

Openness with one's family and other supportive friends is essential, not that they should or will decide on the treatment you undertake, but rather to assist you in arriving at the choices you make.

No one likes to believe that he will ever have to face the choice of treatment for a recurring prostate cancer. Unfortunately, as the Partin Tables illustrate, prostate cancer does have a tendency to reoccur. If there is a single problem I have with the media when reporting on famous men who have been diagnosed and treated for prostate cancer, it is the tendency to state "the disease was caught and 'so-and-so' should recover completely." Certainly everyone hopes and prays that such media reports turn out to be correct. Nonetheless this form of reporting does a gross disservice to men and to the public at large. Prostate cancer is still not totally understood. The usual standard often quoted for cancer patients that "if you survive five years you are probably cured," is generally not applicable for prostate cancer patients. Most men if, they did nothing, statistically survive five years from the time of initial diagnosis. I am now over six years from initial diagnosis. I consider that I am now entering the critical stage in my history of my prostate cancer. I will feel that I am cured only as I cross over the 10 to 15 year mark. I cannot help but reflect on my own family history where my mother was treated for breast cancer and survived 8 years before it reoccurred.

The final choices for treatment if the prostate cancer returns are not as limited as they were a short time ago. The rules are the same at this stage as when you were initially diagnosed, namely, make your decision to treat or not, and thereafter do not have any regrets. Experimental programs are reported almost every month addressing reoccurring malignancy of all types and prostate cancer is no different in this regard. How effective any of these test or protocol programs may be is difficult to assess in the short range. Further, if the program is part of protocol you may not know if you have received the drug or a placebo.

PART IV

CONCLUSION

Summary Remarks

In keeping with my plan when I starting writing this book, I have attempted to omit my own personal views concerning the treatment options. I did not desire to sway any reader, or create the impression that I had found the perfect treatment solution. The treatment I selected was for myself. I determined that it provided the best for my medical and psychological needs. It worked for me and regardless of the side effects I endured. I would not have undertaken a different approach if given the chance to do it over. This book was never intended to be "my story." The need to provide men some understanding of the nature of the disease and the options currently available transcends any one person's experiences.

There is an important lesson to be learned, nonetheless, from my own experience in selecting a particular treatment modality. Prior to my research, I had a general distaste at the thought of surgery to correct the problem. Parts of my beliefs were predicated upon my experience with my mother, who had undergone horrendous surgery during her lifetime, complete with pain and disfigurement. Like most men, beneath it all there was a degree of cowardice that also had me looking for reasonable alternatives. Perhaps the most difficult problems I encountered were the apparent contradictions, disagreements, and professional preferences amongst supposed experts in the field. Who was I to believe? How could I as a layman make an informed choice that was reasonable and effective for my condition? Was I competent to cut through the professional stubbornness to evaluate my correct course of action? How much time did I have to both investigate and arrive at appropriate conclusions. From diagnosis to final treatment for my prostate cancer would span eleven months.

The first step I undertook was to recognize that prostate cancer, unlike many other malignancies, was not going to kill me in within the next week. I had been diagnosed with a prostate cancer by biopsy alone. The amount of cancer discovered was less then 5% of the gross sample. The Gleason Score was a mid-range 6, although the PSA was a relatively high 13.5, with the subsequent PSA II test at 16.5 with the free radical at 14%. My MRI appeared normal in that the pelvic lymph nodes appeared to be grossly clear. My CAT Scan appeared normal. My bone scan gave me a slight scare in that it showed every damage I had ever inflicted upon my body. There were far more damaged and "old" bones then even I imagined. The initial reading of the bone scan stated that two spots on my ribs were "consistent with the spread of prostate cancer." It took three radiologists to finally conclude that this was not the case. With all this information in hand, I took a deep breath and started to seek out as much intelligent information as I could secure. I must state that I did not like most of the information uncovered that was directed at the layman. Medical writers believe the average patient is somewhere between cave dweller and monkey, write much of the available information. No insult intended for the Cave Dweller or the Monkey! There was either not enough information to enable me to make any intelligent decision or information in a highly medically technical format. I needed to find medical information from the professional not necessarily engaged in urology. Although I recognized that I would encounter difficulty with the technical aspects of the data I accessed, it would provide a starting point. I went to Public Library and found little information. My next recourse was the Internet.

The Internet provided me with "data overload." Considerable information was too dated to make me comfortable. Any information before 1996 I disregarded. I made this decision because the entire field of prostate cancer and its treatment is in a state of flux. New information and studies come out almost on a daily basis. The long-term effects of newer treatments are beginning to develop sound statistical foundations. I wanted to know what was the present state of the art. For example, not long ago research conducted at the UCLA Johnson Cancer Center discovered that when a specific gene PTEN mutated it appeared to act as a "gate" which allows growth signals to set prostate cancer into motion. Obviously, if a discovery could be made of how this gate works and how to shut it down when it mutates, prostate cancer might be prevented. The future may well allow the drug industry to develop and design drugs that block the mechanism that is the pathway for the rapid growth of cells leading to prostate cancer. Perhaps drugs are already being tested along with gene therapy, but I decided that I could not wait to see what would develop. Treatment options that were too new, albeit interesting had to be put on the back shelf. I concluded that these new experimental options were not for me.

The amount of information I uncovered worldwide was immense. I decided to narrow the data down into various categories and to see whether there were any common threads that flowed through the topics. Once I found these threads, I was able to narrow the search further. Armed with the information, I was now in a position to direct more telling questions to the urologist and the radiation oncologist. I was troubled by some of the literature that younger men with early stage prostate cancer should have surgery. Further statements indicating that even young men who had localized spread were not candidates for surgery confused this information. Articles and studies indicated in the latter situation patients should be treated with hormone therapy and radiation. Subsequent discussions with physicians made it clear to me that there are no guarantees of cure for early stage prostate cancer, regardless of the therapy undertaken.

The decision, I considered valid for my needs, was seed implantation with 3-D Conformal Beam Radiation, along with hormone therapy to reduce the size of the gland. This seemed to be the least invasive procedure and appeared to offer the best opportunity for long range survival without the side effects of incontinence and impotence. I was to subsequently learn that even with the best medical care and the most meticulous of research, there are no guarantees that you will not fall into the statistical minority and encounter side effects. These bodies we occupy and tend to disregard until some tragedy occurs have a way of reacting on their own terms. Mine has and continues to do so! I have endured all of the side effects I had sought to avoid! From June until early December, I sustained a bout of "urge incontinence" which went round the clock. During the early period of this trauma, I also suffered from intense sharp pain and discomfort while urinating. Every hour or two, I became a worshipper of the porcelain throne! As this problem alleviated, rectal irritation developed. This intensified requiring me to secure a colonoscopy in an attempt to ascertain what was happening to my system. The colonoscopy came back with negative results, although it did indicate some rectal irritation. The gastroenterologist does not believe that the irritation is radiation related. The urologist and the radiologist believed that this was not an uncommon side effect of radiation therapy and in fact could have occurred even years after the radiation had ceased to be active in the body. This form of conflict of opinions between physicians is something I have come to accept during the treatment for my prostate cancer although fortunately, more often then not my treating physicians have been in agreement. All of the side effects finally ceased and all in all have faded into the dim recesses of my memory of the events.

The final problem I have encountered has been the onset of partial impotence. My urologist has suggested that I consider "Vitamin V—Viagra," or more recently, Cialis. The problem has shown signs of improving with nocturnal erections returning, although the level of sensation is not what it had been prior to my treatments.

None of these problems were supposed to have occurred. Most individuals who have undergone my treatment have not sustained any of these side effects. I have been informed that in all probability all of these problems will end, as did the urge incontinence. Every three months since the end of my formal treatment I have had PSA tests. The results of the four tests have been in order of first to last: 0.00; 0.13; 0.0; 0.16. Then suddenly the next test result was 0.26 followed by two years of 0.3 every six months until the test in July 2004 which came back as 0.2. The lower PSA has continued with the February 2005 result being 0.21. In June 2005 my PSA continued at 0.21. I am certain by the time the book has been published there will have been another test. The PSA will fluctuate, and I have been informed that as long as it stays under 0.5 the treatment will be deemed successful. Nonetheless there are studies that indicate that the risk of reoccurrence is statistically higher if after radiation treatment the PSA does not stabilize out at 0.2 or less. Did I have apprehension as I noted the rise in the PSA? Intellectually, I could have argued that statistically the results have been consistent. The first test indicates that I still had the hormones in my system. The subsequent tests certainly are far superior to my pre treatment levels of 13.5 and 16.5. I have a long path to still tread.

In spite of all of these problems, I have followed my own advice. I have not looked back nor do I regret the decision I have made for the treatment path I have undertaken. I can be master of my destiny only up to a certain extent. My body will be the final arbiter of what it will or will not do. Like all men involved with the sudden realization that they have prostate cancer, I must learn to live each day with the potential and the promise to remain steadfast regardless of what may come my way. I cannot become obsessive, but must come to terms with my pathology. My life must continue with the hope that I will be one of the seventy percent who have defeated the disease. If I am not so fortunate, I hope that new and more aggressive weapons will be available to me to continue the fight. Each day brings with it both opportunity and challenge. Prostate cancer is just one of many challenges that I face in my life.

What prostate cancer has shown me is that I am not alone in my struggle. Millions of men have and will continue to face the challenge of this uniquely male disease. I have learned to take command of my own destiny to every extent possible. Although physicians have become my partners in the struggle, I remain the master of my ship. I must navigate through the troubled waters taking into account the whole "me." Prostate cancer affects the whole man, his spouse, or significant other. Concern for quality of life is as much a part of how you confront the cancer as is the treatment of the cancer itself.

There was another aspect of the diagnosis of prostate cancer that forced me to address the image I had of myself as a man. What was important to me? Who was I? Men as a group in the United States especially, have been weaned upon the milk of "machismo." In a post World War II society of sexual liberation and the "Marlboro Man," prowess has been the model for many men. Nothing therefore challenges a man more than the sudden fear of the loss of his virility. This becomes more of a problem when the man is still young enough to be sexually active. American men tend also not to be open and not to discuss, even with their physicians, issues of sexual dysfunction. Although Viagra has started to make a small dent into this wall of silence, it is not a topic of conversation that at the time of my procedure was often heard in mixed polite company. Clearly the climate has changed today with ads on prime time television for Viagra, Levitra and Cialis. I suspect as new drugs are developed more publicity will be heard. The thrust of advertising these drugs today is not so much aimed at erectile dysfunction, but rather as a life style enhancement.

While awaiting my seed implantation, I confronted this sense of discomfort, when I engaged in conversation a gentleman in the next bed awaiting a different procedure. The casual talk centered about why we were in Day Surgery and who were our treating physicians. Upon hearing that we both used the same urologist, I was informed what a great person the physician was and how successful he had been in performing surgery on him. Further small talk revealed my prostate cancer, as did this gentleman's. Undaunted by my imminent implantation, I asked whether or not he had had any side effects from his prostate cancer surgery. An emphatic "none," was the reply coupled with a wink that "everything was working fine!" Only when he was moved for his hernia operation did his wife disclose he had continual incontinence but that Viagra wasn't working. I am convinced that our mutual physician was not aware of these problems. This has always been a source of concern, having no such personal hesitation to raise issues to my physicians, how many men die or suffer without adequate relief due to pride, ego, and silence?

It is because of these attitudes that it is so essential loved ones are brought into the entire process of the prostate cancer scenario from diagnosis through treatment and thereafter. Spouses, significant others, and friends all share a profound nexus to what you are going through. Starting with my first blood test indicating an elevated PSA, I sat down with my wife and a dear older friend (who incidentally was also a psychiatrist) in order to discuss what had just descended upon my life. Although I never have considered myself cancer phobic, I needed more. I needed to know that I had a support group with whom I could discuss my feelings and my search for a decision for treatment. I did have some knowledge of prostate problems. I had witnessed my father-in-law undergo surgery for the removal of his prostate and I knew what side effects he had encountered even though his was a benign condition.

Once the second biopsy had confirmed the presence of prostate cancer, all subsequent decisions and discussions with potential treating physicians, research into treatments, where and when to commence treatment, involved my family and close friends. It was also so important to have someone present when I had discussions with potential treating physicians. Having an individual present to listen to what is being said is absolutely critical to your decisional process. Critical hearing is as vital as asking the right questions I discussed earlier in the book.

My diagnosing physician appeared to me to disparage any treatment other then radical surgery. He also indicated that surgery would "cure me!" I was personally convinced that I hadn't either heard correctly or I was perhaps reading into what was said. Only when my wife confirmed the comments did I realize that what I believed had been stated was correct. Unfortunately, the diagnosing physician who pushed so hard for surgery himself shortly thereafter died of prostate cancer. He had had surgery at a leading medical center some years before. I point out this fact not to dissuade any man from surgery but rather to illustrate that prostate cancer can be unpredictable even for the experts who confront it on a daily basis.

When I went for a second opinion at another major medical center in New York City, my favorite psychiatrist came along. I have often felt that this friend could not believe, as a medical professional, some of what I had been indicating to him about my prior experiences with his colleague at the institution with which he was associated. He came along not only as an accommodation to me but also I suspect to be able to inform me that I was in fact crazy! He learned that not only was this not the case, but that he would serve to reinforce my understanding of what I had been experiencing from various physicians.

My second opinion re-diagnosed the Gleason Score I had received and indicated that surgery was my only chance for survival. Using the Partin

Table, I was further told that even with surgery there would be a 40% chance of a reoccurrence. Only time will ultimately tell who was right.

In the June 28th 2000 edition of the Journal of the American Medical Association an article appeared comparing treatment recommendations between radiation oncologists and urologists for the treatment of clinically localized prostate cancer. Although almost five and one half years have passed since my last treatment here again in this prestigious Journal, I encountered the same disagreements between specialists as I had faced when first seeking answers to what treatment I believed would serve my purposes. What continues to be even more frustrating is the lack of any major studies or even discussions relating to combined therapies. Every article, including the June 28th Journal discussion, paints the treatment therapy in "either or terms." Nowhere in the discussion was any talk about hormone therapy coupled with external beam radiation coupled with brachytherapy. In analyzing hormone therapy there is also no mention of combined hormone therapies utilizing different hormones at the same time. The comfort level of the specialist appears to dictate what treatment is suggested to the patient.

Talking through the treatment options with others helps to focus your comfort level. Even though friends may not be experts and may possess the same level of ignorance concerning prostate cancer, they do provide psychological reinforcement. Remember that in the end the treatment option you select must be yours.

Other diseases have effects on family and friends, but prostate cancer operates on the psychosexual level. The fear of the loss of ones' manhood can be overwhelming. The need to recognize that a normal life need not end with a diagnosis of prostate cancer requires open communication and collective support.

There is a single warning that must be recognized. If the closest of family and friends are cancer phobic, you need to assure them that in most cases of early diagnosis of prostate cancer you are not in imminent danger of dying—even if you choose no treatment whatsoever. Prostate cancer is everyone's business. Mutual support and knowledge are essential to achieve good long-term results both physically as well as psychologically. Perhaps equally important is to insulate yourself from the sometimes constant bombardment of others who "knew someone with the disease and was treated by...." Well meaning people can confuse and scare without intending to do so. The decisions that you make must be reasonable and done with understanding that everyone is essentially different. What may work for one individual, both physically and mentally, may not be the way to deal with the disease insofar as your case is concerned. When you finally arrive at the right decision for treatment for you, never look back!

My decisions pertaining to my prostate cancer are perhaps best summed up in the words of William Shakespeare, "to thine own self be true, then thou canst be false to any man!"

PART V

REFERENCE MATERIAL

Websites

(World Wide Web—Internet)

The following is a very selective list of Internet Web Sites that possess information of interest to the prostate cancer patient. This list is not intended to be all-inclusive of the vast data available on the Internet. In the process of attempting to secure information, I became increasingly aware of "salesmanship" as well as old information that no longer has significant credibility. I do not refer to any sites that are more than two years old. I do not refer to sites from local medical practices that are advertisements for their offices. Rather, I have limited the web sites to major sources such as governmental study centers and major medical institutions without attempting to be overly limiting in providing access to the broadest spectrum of data.

http//www. Prostatehealth.com

http//www.prostatecancer.com

http//www.cancernet.nci.nih.gov/soa/Prostate_cancer_Physician

http//www.prostatecancer.on.ca

http//www.cancerresearch.org/prostate.html

http//pcaw.com

http//www.pslgroup.com/PROSTATECANCER.html

http//www.cinenet-prostate/awareness/

http//www.cornmed,com/Prostate/Screening-EarlyDetection.html

http//www.medsch.wisc.edu/pca/faq/radiation.html

http//www.4npcc.org/

http//www.biostat.wisc.edu/html

http//www.imsddmeb.unibonnde/cancernet/101229.html

http//www.prostate-cancer.org.uk

http//www.prostate.com

http//webmdcorn/topic_summary/1452/327

Once you have commenced looking through the above web sites it will become very apparent how many different locations exist containing information about prostate cancer, its' causes and its' treatment. It is extremely easy to find yourself in a situation of "information overload!"

Be careful in whatever research you undertake on the Internet. The fact is that the various medical centers do have prejudices concerning the treatment for prostate cancer. There are deriding comments about any treatment other then surgery from some medical institutions and their staff. The published data from these sources on the Internet must be weighed against the totality of information you have collected. Beware of any

Internet site that promises a definite "cure" through one procedure or another. Look at the date of the data presented by each site you may visit.

Information more then two years old is already subject to further examination. The more recent the dates of the data presented, and the more current the statistics, the better chance you have for arriving at an intelligent assessment. Remember that there is new information being presented on prostate cancer almost on a weekly basis. The best example of this fact is the announcement in April of 2000, that a new test for prostate cancer is being investigated which will look for a certain enzyme in the urine. The researchers believe this test will provide an earlier detection of the presence of prostate cancer then the traditional blood test administered to arrive at PSA levels. In and of itself the PSA level does not prove the existence of cancer in the prostate.

Whatever research you conduct on the Internet make certain to print out copies of the data you feel you may need to review at some subsequent period. The printed copy will also be of benefit to you should you desire to ask your physician about any facts contained in these reports.

Organizations

There are numerous organizations concerned with the issue of prostate cancer and the effect it has on those diagnosed with the disease as well as family members. Some of these organizations are "local" and some are "umbrella" groups that either contain several other organizations or provide access to local support agencies. The list set forth is by no means all-inclusive. Your local hospital, physician, or chapter of the American Cancer Society can be very helpful in providing the names, addresses and phone numbers of local support groups. Many individuals do not feel at ease within support groups and are hesitant to talk to others about their fears, doubts and needs. Yet, in many ways support groups provide a very useful service if for no other reason then they indicate that you are not alone with your problem. As more publicity has been available about prostate cancer through newspaper articles and television discussions, the numbers and availability of support groups will undoubtedly grow in numbers and convenience.

Whether you choose to involve yourself in any of these groups is ultimately up to you. Recognize however, that prostate cancer is not your disease alone. The disease and its' treatment will affect everyone around you, be it your spouse or significant other. These individuals are a part of your life and will feel your anxieties, your shifting moods and will endure them with you as you undergo your treatments. These individuals may need support along with you in to better understand the nature of the disease and the outlook for you before and after treatment. What I have discovered is that my learning experience made me a teacher of those close to me. Do not shut your loved ones out of the process!

1. The National Prostate Cancer Coalition
1156 15th Street NW, Suite 905
Washington, DC 20005
(202) 463-9455

2. The American Prostate Society
1340F Charwood Road
Hanover, MD 21076
(410) 859-9455

3. CaP Cure
1250 Fourth Street, Suite 360
Santa Monica, CA 90401
(310) 458-2873

4. Prostate Cancer Support Network
1218 North Charles Street
Baltimore, MD 21201
(800) 828-7866

5. US-TOO International
930 North York Road, Suite 50
Hinsdale, IL 60521
(630) 323-1002

6. Cancer Care Inc.
1180 Avenue of the Americas
New York, NY 10036
(212) 221-3300

7. American Cancer Society
1599 Clifton Road North East
Atlanta, GA 30329
(800) 227-2345

8. National Cancer Institute
Office of Cancer Communications,
National Cancer Institute
Building 31, Room 10A16
Bethesda, MD 20892
(800) 422-6237

9. The Wellness Community
2716 Ocean Park Boulevard, Suite 1040
Santa Monica, CA 90405
(310) 314-2555
10. American Foundation for Urologic Disease
300 West Pratt Street, Suite 400
Baltimore, MD 21201
(800) 242-2383

11. Prostate Cancer Research and Education Foundation
6699 Alvaro Road, Suite 2301
San Diego, CA 92120
(619) 287-8860

12. International Cancer Alliance
4853 Cordell Avenue, Suite II
Bethesda, MD 20814
(301) 654-793

The above list does not indicate any preference or support on my part for these organizations over others that may exist. The organizations listed are readily available to the patient and provide a good starting point from which to seek other groups. For patients in Canada, the following address is for a national umbrella organization for prostate cancer organizations throughout the country and will enable Canadian patients to find support groups across the nation.

13. The Canadian Prostate Cancer Network
The National Association of Prostate Cancer Support Groups
Post Office Box 1253
Lakefield, ON, K0L 2H0, Canada
Fax: (705) 652-0663

Similar organizations can be found for most nations in the western world. Great Britain has several, as does the European Community. Most of these organizations can lead you to other groups. There are plenty of support organizations available.

Together with the Web Sites provided in the previous section, the patient should be able to secure data sufficient to your needs. Always remember being a well-informed patient puts you in the best position to assist in your own treatment!

The Partin Tables

The Partin Tables divide predictions of the cancer penetrating the Capsule of the prostate gland based upon the PSA level detected, Gleason Score, and the Stage of the disease that the pathologist has determined for the particular patient. Any change in these three factors will effect the percentage probabilities.

Prediction of Probability of Established Capsular Penetration (%)
PSA = 0.0-4.0 ng/ml

Gleason Score	Stage T1a	Stage T1b	Stage T1c	Stage T2a	Stage T2b	Stage T2c	Stage T3a
2-4	9	19	10	18	25	21	—
5	17	32	18	30	40	34	51
6	19	35	21	34	43	37	53
7	—	44	31	45	51	45	52
8-10	—	43	34	47	48	42	—

It is very important to remember that the above and following percentages are "probability predictions." As increasing numbers of men are diagnosed with prostate cancer, the statistical probabilities may or may not change. Even if the cancer has penetrated the capsule, either surgery or external conformal beam radiation may eliminate any further spread of the disease. Coupled with the problem of under-diagnosis or misdiagnosis of the disease, the Partin Statistical Tables may not be accurate as an aid in arriving at your prognosis. As discussed in this book, prostate cancer has a mind of its' own and no two men's condition are exactly the same.

Prediction of Probability of Established Capsular Penetration (%)
PSA = 4.1-10.0 ng/ml

Gleason Score	Stage T1a	Stage T1b	Stage T1c	Stage T2a	Stage T2b	Stage T2c	Stage T3a
2-4	14	27	15	26	35	29	44
5	25	42	27	41	50	43	57
6	27	44	30	44	52	46	57
7	36	48	40	52	54	48	48
8-10	34	42	40	49	46	40	34

The following two charts involve PSA levels that are considered high enough to alter the statistical probability of long term survival.

Prediction of Probability of Established Capsular Penetration (%)
PSA = 10.1-20 ng/ml

Gleason Score	Stage T1a	Stage T1b	Stage T1c	Stage T2a	Stage T2b	Stage T2c	Stage T3a
2-4	20	36	22	35	43	37	—
5	33	50	35	50	57	51	59
6	—	49	38	52	57	50	54
7	38	46	45	55	51	45	40
8-10	—	33	40	46	38	33	26

Prediction of Probability of Established Capsular Penetration (%)
PSA = > 20.0 ng/ml

Gleason Score	Stage T1a	Stage T1b	Stage T1c	Stage T2a	Stage T2b	Stage T2c	Stage T3a
2-4	—	47	34	48	52	—	—
5	—	57	48	60	61	55	54
6	—	51	49	60	57	51	46
7	—	—	46	51	43	37	29
8-10	—	24	34	37	28	23	17

Illustrations

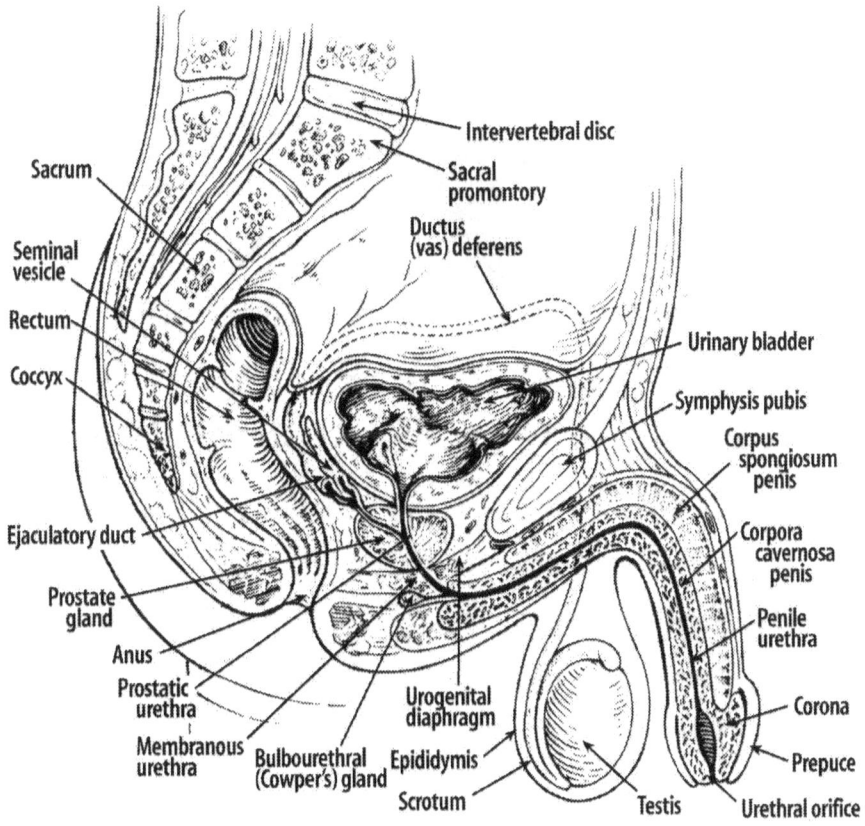

Intervertebral disc

Sacrum

Sacral promontory

Ductus (vas) deferens

Seminal vesicle

Rectum

Coccyx

Urinary bladder

Symphysis pubis

Corpus spongiosum penis

Ejaculatory duct

Corpora cavernosa penis

Prostate gland

Penile urethra

Anus

Prostatic urethra

Corona

Membranous urethra

Urogenital diaphragm

Bulbourethral (Cowper's) gland

Epididymis

Prepuce

Scrotum

Testis

Urethral orifice

Figure 1: The territory

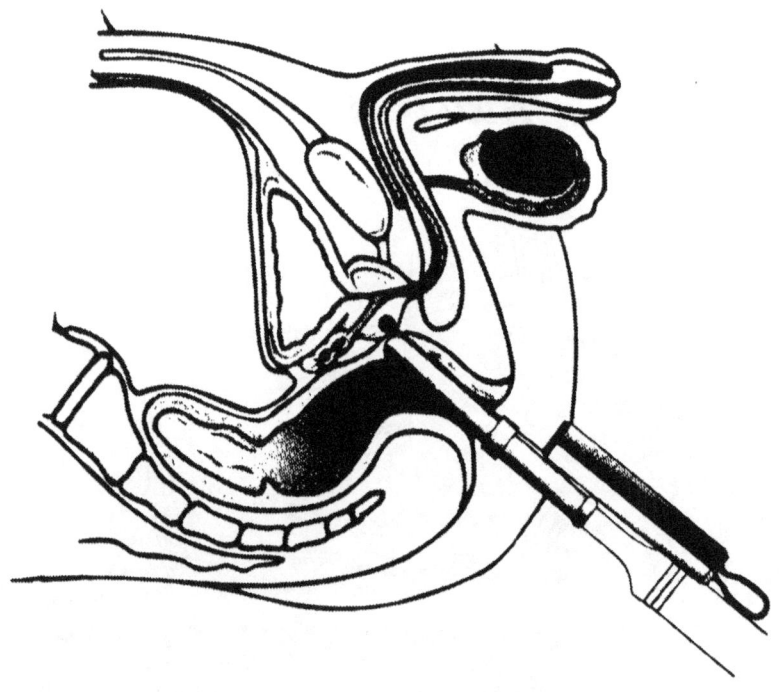

Figure 2: Transrectal Ultrasound Prostate Biopsy

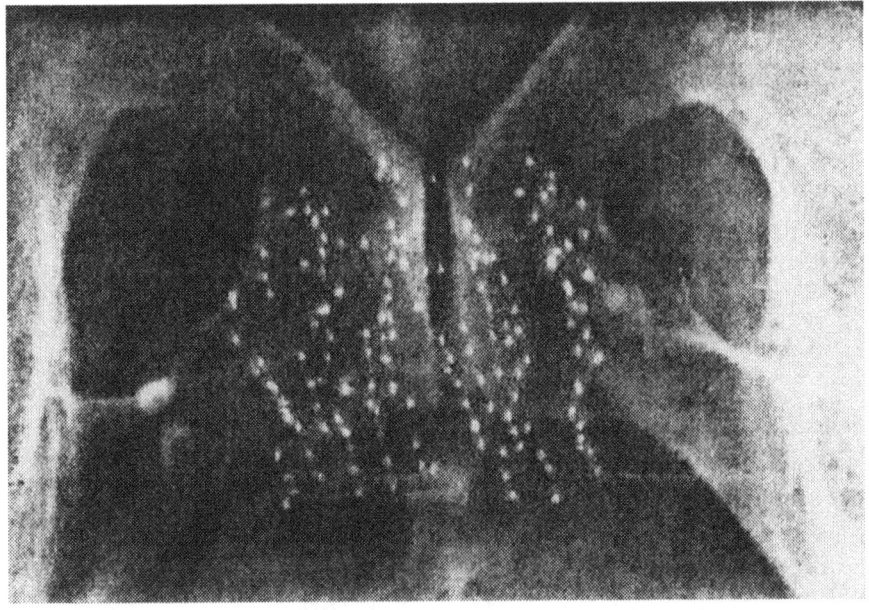

Figure 3: Brachytherapy

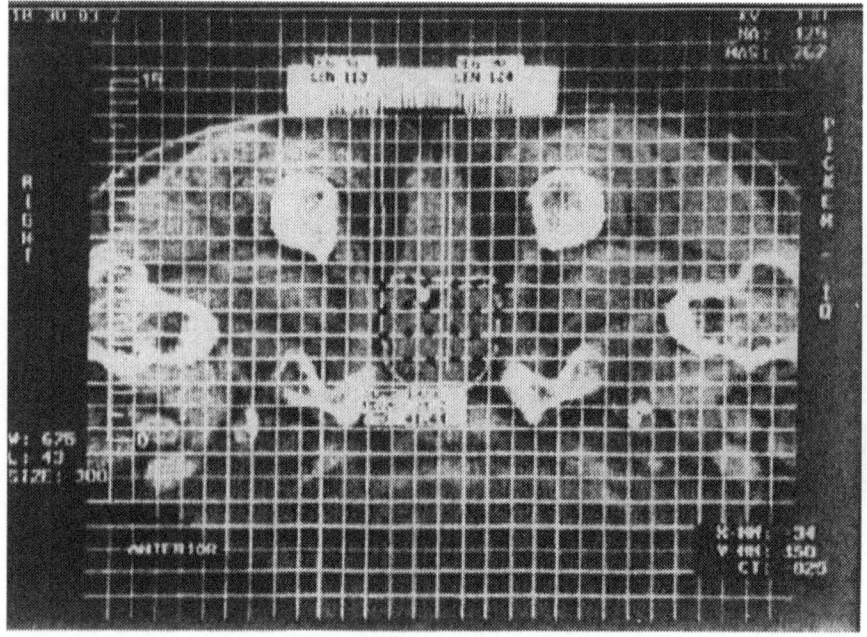

Figure 4: Brachytherapy
This figure shows the "grid" pattern used by the Dosimitrist to place the seeds

The Gleason Grading System

The progression goes from 1 to 5 with 5 being the most serious.

Grade 1 - Round glands - Well defined - Together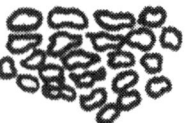

Grade 2 - Round glands - Not together - Vague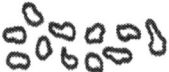

Grade 3A - Irregular shape and spacing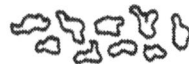

Grade 3B - Small Glands - No chains or chords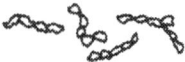

Grade 3C - Rounded and smooth cylinders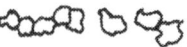

Grade 4A - Glands fused into chains and cords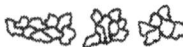

Grade 4B - Many large clear cells

Grade 5A - Solid Sheets, single cells or nests

Grade 5B - Ragged sheets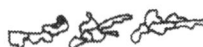

Figure 5

Glossary

The following words and their definitions are referenced within the book. This is not intended to be a complete list of terms you may encounter in research pertaining to prostate cancer.

Abdomen: the area from underneath the rib cage to the pelvic region.

Actin: a protein essential to allowing cancer cells to break free from the prostate gland and escape to surrounding tissue.

Adenocarcinoma: typically, the cancer most commonly found in the prostate.

Adrenal glands: located on the top of the kidneys. The adrenal glands also produce sex hormones.

Androgen: produced in both the testicles and the adrenal glands, a hormone that creates the typical male characteristics.

Anti-androgen: a drug whose purpose is to interfere with the body's ability to use the androgen hormone. An example would be the drug Casodex.

BPH: Benign Prostatic Hyperplasia is a common condition of male aging where the prostate gland enlarges and tends to create difficulties in urination.

Bilateral: as referenced in this book, the two sides of the prostate gland.

Biopsy: the removal of a sample of tissue that is later examined by a pathologist in order to ascertain whether cancer or some other disease is present.

Bladder: located above the prostate, it is the organ that holds and stores urine, allowing it to pass through the urethra out of the body.

Bone Scan: utilizing an injection of a radioactive substance that is taken up by the skeleton. In the event of the spread of cancer, it enables the physician to identify the location of secondary invasions.

Brachytherapy: a treatment for prostate cancer where either Iodine or Palladium radioactive seeds are injected into the prostate to destroy the cancer.

Capsule: the prostate gland is contained within a flexible cellular structure, which defines the size and shape of the gland.

Casodex: the trade name for an anti-androgen to block the body's ability to use testosterone.

CAT SCAN: a diagnostic technique where a computerized imaging system allows the physician to create three-dimensional and cross sectional images of a portion of the body.

Catheter: commonly used by urologists, it is a flexible tube inserted into the urethra and into the bladder to enable urine to drain freely. Sometimes called a "Foley."

Cowper Glands: sometimes referred to as "bulbourethral glands," these empty into the base of the penis. They secrete a mucous fluid and are part of the fluid portion of the semen.

Cryosurgery: the injection of usually liquid nitrogen into the prostate in order to kill off the gland and any cancerous cells.

Cystoscope: a device utilized by urologists who insert it into the urethra to provide them with a view of the urethra and bladder.

DNA: the structure that carries the genetic code within each cell of the human body.

Dosimetrist: an individual responsible for calculating the dosage of radiation to be given to a patient.

DRE: digital rectal examination; performed by a physician by inserting a finger into the rectum in order to feel the prostate.

Dysuria: painful urination usually caused by BPH or other disorders of the bladder, prostate, or urethra.

Ejaculation: the process of passing semen through the urethra to outside the penis.

Erectile Dysfunction: a situation caused by several factors, including surgery, wherein there is a failure to achieve an erection of the penis.

External Beam Radiation: radiation therapy wherein radiation is delivered to various parts of the body from an outside source and aimed at an internal tumor.

Flow rate: the measurement of the rate and volume of urine passed during urination to assist the urologist in determining whether the urethra may be obstructed as well as the bladder not emptying.

Free radical: utilized to describe substances produced within the human body which tend to damage the DNA of the cells and can lead to the development of cancers.

Gleason Score: a method for determining the different development of the cancerous cells within the prostate. The grading system is used to assist physicians in determining the differences between the normal prostate cells and the malignant ones.

Green tea: used by the Chinese for centuries, green tea is now becoming recognized as a potentially significant factor in the prevention of various types of cancer.

Hormone Therapy: the use of hormones to treat prostate cancer. Traditionally, the hormones utilized seek to lessen both the production of testosterone and to prevent its use by the body.

Incontinence: the inability to control urination. Incontinence can be either urge or stress incontinence. In either situation, the patient can additionally sustain psychological and physical problems.

Interstitial radiation therapy: another name for brachytherapy or internal seed implantation.

Ischiopubic ramus: the structure surrounding the prostate.

Laproscopic lymphhadenectomy: a procedure involving the use of an instrument making a small incision to remove the lymph node in the pelvic region of the body in order to determine whether the prostate cancer has spread.

Lobe: the prostate gland has two sides (lobes). Often, the cancer is localized in only one of the "lobes" of the gland.

Low-grade PIN: a condition many physicians and researchers believe may be an indicator of later onset of prostate cancer as much as twenty or thirty years from the detection of the infection. Sometimes referred to as prostatic intraepithelial neoplasia.

Lupron: a commercially produced luteinizing hormone given to cancer patients in order to interfere with the production of testosterone.

Lycopene: a component of tomatoes and other similar vegetables which is believed to be effective in preventing prostate cancer and slowing the growth of existent prostate cancer.

Lymph nodes: the lymphatic system of the body acts much as a filter for removing the body's harmful bacteria and other toxic materials. Because it also carries various cells which fight diseases, the lymph nodes can become infected themselves. Cancer cells also can be found in the nodes from other parts of the body and indicate a spread of the disease.

Malignant (Malignancy): a term utilized to describe various forms of cancer.

Metastasis: the discovery of a spread of the cancer from its original location to another part of the body, sometimes referred to as a "secondary location."

MRI: Magnetic resonance imaging is a diagnostic tool which enables the physician to produce two and three-dimensional images of the internal portions of the human body. It is one of the diagnostic tools utilized in determining the extent of prostate cancer and whether it has spread.

Monoclonal antibodies: genetically engineered identical cells, sometimes carrying a specific drug utilized to fight a particular disease.

Nanograms per milliliter: the measurement of the amount of prostate specific antigen in the blood stream.

Negative: the indication that a test or tests for the presence of disease such as cancer shows no evidence of the disease.

Nerve sparing: when discussing prostate cancer, describes a surgical procedure where the nerves responsible for erectile function of the penis are preserved when the prostate gland is removed.

Orchiectomy: the removal of the testicles. In the case of prostate cancer, this procedure is often performed when the cancer has spread to prevent the production of testosterone.

Palliative therapy: a treatment which does not cure the patient, but seeks to make the patient more comfortable and to alleviate some of the symptoms.

Partin Co-Efficient Tables: a statistical tool which includes the PSA, Gleason Scores, and biopsy staging results in order to predict whether the prostate cancer has spread beyond the gland.

PC-SPES: a homeopathic compound of eight different herbs that is being studied as a possible control or cure for prostate cancer. Available over the counter, there are potentially dangerous side affects to its use.

Pelvic Lymph Node Dissection: the removal of the pelvic lymph node in order to determine whether the prostate cancer has spread outside of the gland. Sometimes referred to by its initials, PLND.

Penis: the male organ within which the urethra is located, providing an outlet for urine and for the passage of semen during sexual intercourse.

Perineal prostatectomy: the surgical removal of the prostate gland through the perineum region of the body.

Perineum: that portion of the body between the testicular sac (the scrotum) and the anus.

PET Scan: Positron Emission Tomography. A diagnostic technique utilizing a metabolic marker to provide a three dimensional image of the body.

PIN (Prostatic Intraepithelial Neoplasia): see Low Grade PIN.

Prognosis: the potential for the patient's recovery or progression of the disease.

Prostascint: a commercially developed monoclonal antibody that holds promise in the treatment of prostate cancer.

Prostatitis: generalized infection of the urinary tract, which can be bacterial or nonbacterial in nature. This condition can become chronic.

Prostatron: a recently approved device utilized in the treatment of prostate cancer with microwaves.

Prostatectomy: the removal of the prostate gland utilizing surgery through either retropubic or perineal procedures.

Prostatic Intraepithelial Neoplasia: see PIN.

PSA: prostrate specific antigen is a substance secreted by the prostate gland. When the level of PSA is above the normal range of 0.0 to 4.0, or rises rapidly between tests, there is an indication of some problem in the prostate gland. The PSA test is a simple blood test.

PSA II: a relatively recent improvement over the older PSA test, PSA II measures the percentage of "free PSA" found in the blood stream to the total PSA levels. The higher the ratio of free PSA to the total PSA, the less likely that prostate cancer exists.

PTEN: recently discovered gene believed to mutate in men with prostate cancer allowing for uncontrolled malignant growth of cells in the prostate.

Radiation oncology: the medical specialty wherein a physician uses radiation in various forms to treat cancers.

Radiation therapy: the utilization of various forms and types of radiation, both internal and external, for the treatment of diseases such as cancer.

Radical prostatectomy: the total removal of the prostate gland and some of the surrounding supportive functions of the gland, such as the seminal vesicles and the pelvic lymph node.

Rectum: the end of the intestines that terminates in the anus.

Retropubic prostatectomy: the surgical procedure wherein the prostate gland is removed by making an incision in the lower abdomen in order to locate it.

Saw Palmetto: a substance made from a berry, which appears to have a positive affect on the shrinkage of the prostate gland. Available over the counter without prescription, it has been utilized in Europe for several years and recently in the United States.

Scrotum: the sac of skin between the legs of men, which contains the testicles.

Selenium: an element found in some foods that is being investigated as having an affect on the prevention of prostate and other cancers. Selenium in large doses may have toxic side effects.

Semen: the white-to-yellowish fluid that makes up the ejaculate of men. There are several different glands, involving portions of the prostate, and surrounding tissues produce the fluid.

Side effects: reactions to various forms of medicines and treatments, some of which can be potentially dangerous.

Soy Beans: a bean that has been found to contain very powerful antioxidants. Widely grown and used throughout the world, there is more and more proof that diets high in soy are extremely healthy and may fight several forms of cancer, including prostate cancer.

Stage: a term utilized to define the extent of a disease.

Temporary brachytherapy: the temporary implantation of radioactive seeds within the prostate as a treatment for prostate cancer.

Testicles: the two male glands located within the scrotum between the legs of the male. The testicles are the primary source for the production of testosterone.

Testosterone: the basic male hormone, which is essential for the production of sperm and needed for reproduction.

Transrectal Ultrasound (TRUS): through the use of a special instrument called a probe, ultrasound wave lengths are utilized in order to create an image of the prostate.

Transurethral Resection of the Prostate (TURP): a procedure wherein the urologist inserts an instrument through the urethra in order to remove any obstruction of urine flow. Most often used when BPH has put pressure on the urethra, restricting the flow of urine. The prostate gland may be partially surgically removed by this procedure.

Tumor: an irregular, abnormal growth of cells that may disrupt normal function of a part of the body such as an organ or gland. Tumors may be malignant or nonmalignant.

Urethra: the tube that leads from the bladder through the penis, enabling urine and seminal fluids to exit the body.

Urgency: the sensation of having to urinate or defecate immediately. Uncontrollable bladder and rectal movements may accompany it.

Urologist: a specially trained physician who treats disorders of the urinary system.

Vas deferens: the tubes which enable the sperm to go from the testicles to the prostate gland.

Vasectomy: a surgical procedure wherein the vas deferns is cut. This prevents sperm from passing into the prostate and ultimately being ejaculated.

Verumontanum: the prostate gland is divided into three very distinct regions or zones. Within the central region of the prostate are the ejaculation ducts or verumontanum.

Viagra: A prescription drug developed by Pfizer Pharmaceutical to aid in the relief of erectile dysfunction. It is effective for most men although not everyone has success with the drug. There are also serious potential side effects for men with certain heart conditions.

Vitamins: Vitamins such as A, C, D, and E are substances that the body utilizes to maintain cellular and general health. In recent years, these substances have been investigated more and more in order to determine if they can play a significant role in the prevention of disease.

X-Rays: a diagnostic tool used to make images of the internal portions of the human body through the use of a form of radiation.

Zinc: a mineral found in low levels in some foods and thought to be essential for good health and proper prostate function.

Zoladex: like Lupron, a commercially produced luteinizing hormone utilized in the treatment of prostate cancer.

978-0-595-24337-2
0-595-24337-1